The Effective Management of
Renal Cell Carcinoma

Titles of related interest in the UK Key Advances in Clinical Practice Series

SOLID TUMOURS
The Effective Management of Malignant Melanoma
The Effective Management of Ovarian Cancer, 1st, 2nd and 3rd edns
The Effective Management of Lung Cancer, 1st, 2nd and 3rd edns
The Effective Management of Colorectal Cancer, 1st, 2nd, 3rd and 4th edns
The Effective Management of Breast Cancer, 1st and 2nd edns
The Effective Management of Prostatic Cancer
The Effective Management of Renal Cell Cancer

HAEMATOLOGICAL MALIGNANCIES
The Effective Management of Non-Hodgkin's Lymphoma, 1st and 2nd edns
The Effective Prevention and Management of Systemic Fungal Infection in Haematological
Malignancy, 1st and 2nd edns
The Effective Management of Common Complications of Induction Chemotherapy in
Haematological Malignancy
The Effective Management of Chronic Lymphocytic Leukaemia
The Effective Management of Urological Malignancies

SYMPTOM CONTROL
The Effective Management of Cancer Pain, 1st and 2nd edns
The Effective Prevention and Control of Symptoms in Cancer

HEALTH POLICY
NICE, CHI and the NHS Reforms: Enabling excellence or imposing control?
Clinical Governance and the NHS Reforms: Enabling excellence or imposing control?
Managed Care Networks: Principles and practice

The Effective Management of
Renal Cell Carcinoma

Edited by

Michael Aitchison MD FRCS FRCSUrol
*Consultant Urological Surgeon, Department of Urology, Gartnavel General Hospital,
North Glasgow University Hospitals NHS Trust, Glasgow*

R Tim D Oliver MD FRCP
Sir Joseph Maxwell Professor in Medical Oncology, St Bartholomew's Hospital, London, UK

Andrew Miles MSc MPhil PhD
*Professor of Public Health Sciences &
Editor-in-Chief, Journal of Evaluation in Clinical Practice,
Barts and The London,
Queen Mary's School of Medicine and Dentistry,
University of London, UK*

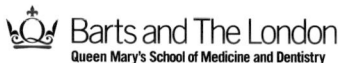

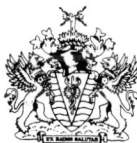

Barts and The London
Queen Mary's School of Medicine and Dentistry

The Royal College
of
Radiologists

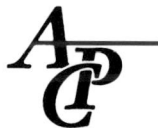

Association
of
Cancer Physicians

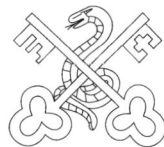

British Association
of
Urological Surgeons

AESCULAPIUS MEDICAL PRESS
LONDON SAN FRANCISCO SYDNEY

Published by

Aesculapius Medical Press (London, San Francisco, Sydney)
PO Box LB48, London EC1A 1LB, UK

British Library Cataloguing in Publication Data
A CIP catalogue record for this book is available from the British Library

ISBN: 1 903044 31 6

While the advice and information in this book are believed to be true and accurate at the
time of going to press, neither the authors nor the publishers nor the sponsoring institutions
can accept any legal responsibility or liability for errors or omissions that may be made.
In particular (but without limiting the generality of the preceding disclaimer) every effort
has been made to check drug usages; however, it is possible that errors have been missed.
Furthermore, dosage schedules are constantly being revised and new side effects recognised.
For these reasons, the reader is strongly urged to consult the drug companies' printed
instructions before administering any of the drugs recommended in this book.

Further copies of this volume are available from:

Claudio Melchiorri
Aesculapius Medical Press
PO Box LB48, Mount Pleasant Mail Centre, Farringdon Road, London EC1A 1LB, UK

Fax: 020 8525 8661
Email: claudio@keyadvances4.demon.co.uk

Typeset, printed and bound in Britain
Peter Powell Origination & Print Limited

Contents

Contributors

Michael Aitchison MD FRCS FRCS(Urol), Consultant Urological Surgeon and Honorary Clinical Senior Lecturer, Department of Urology, Gartnavel General Hospital, North Glasgow University Hospitals NHS Trust, Glasgow

Naomi E Allen MSc DPhil, Research Scientist, Cancer Research UK Epidemiology Unit, University of Oxford

Emma Bromwich MRCS, Specialist Registrar in Urology, Department of Urology, Gartnavel General Hospital, North Glasgow University Hospitals NHS Trust, Glasgow

Paul Cool MD MMedSc(Res) FRCS(Ed) FRCS(Orth), Consultant Orthopaedic and Oncological Surgeon, The Robert Jones and Agnes Hunt Orthopaedic Hospital, Oswestry

Harry Daniels BSc PhD, Professor of Special Education and Educational Psychology, School of Education, University of Birmingham, Birmingham

Jan Derry PhD MSc DCC BSc PGCE, Lecturer in Education, Institute of Education, University of London

Theodora Foukaneli MRCP, Clinical Research Fellow in Haematology, Department of Haematology, St George's Hospital Medical School, London

Martin E Gore PhD FRCP, Professor of Cancer Medicine, The Royal Marsden Hospital, London

Mel F Grainger MB ChB FRCS(Orth), Specialist Registrar in Trauma and Orthopaedics, Department of Spinal Surgery, Royal Orthopaedic Hospital, Birmingham

Viviane Hess MD, Specialist Registrar in Medical Oncology, The Royal Marsden Hospital, London

Alexander J Howie MD FRCPath, Reader in Renal Pathology, University of Birmingham, Birmingham

Nicholas D James MBBS BSc PhD FRCR FRCP, Professor of Clinical Oncology, CRC Institute for Cancer Studies, University of Birmingham and Queen Elizabeth Hospital, Birmingham

Gareth E Jones MB ChB FRCS(Urol), Specialist Registrar in Urology, Scottish Lithotriptor Centre, Western General Hospital, Edinburgh

Julian E Kabala MRCP FRCR, Consultant Radiologist, Bristol Royal Infirmary, Bristol

Andrew M McGee MB ChB FRCS, Specialist Registrar in Trauma and Orthopaedics, Department of Spinal Surgery, Royal Orthopaedic Hospital, Birmingham

Eamonn R Maher BSc MD FRCP, Professor of Medical Genetics and Head, Section of Medical and Molecular Genetics, Department of Paediatrics and Child Health, University of Birmingham, and West Midlands Regional Genetics Service, Birmingham

Agnieszka Michael MRCP, Clinical Research Fellow in Medical Oncology, Department of Oncology, St George's Hospital Medical School, London

R Tim D Oliver MD FRCP, Sir Joseph Maxwell Professor in Medical Oncology, St Bartholomew's Hospital, London

Vincent J O'Neill MD BSc MRCP, Clinical Lecturer, Beatson Oncology Centre, Glasgow

Hardev S Pandha PhD MRCP FRACP, Senior Lecturer in Medical Oncology, Department of Oncology, St George's Hospital Medical School, London

James Patton FRCS(Tr) FRCS(Orth), Specialist Registrar, Royal Orthopaedic Hospital Birmingham, Birmingham

Rubina Rahman BSc, Research Associate, School of Education, University of Birmingham, Birmingham

Sarah Richards MB ChB MRCS, Surgical Research Registrar, University of Bristol and Urology Department, Gloucestershire Royal Hospital, Gloucester

Alastair WS Ritchie FRCS, Consultant Urological Surgeon, Gloucestershire Royal Hospital, Gloucester

Scott Sommerville FRCS(Orth), Oncology Fellow, Royal Orthopaedic Hospital Birmingham, Birmingham

Alistair J Stirling FRCS, Consultant Spinal Surgeon, Department of Spinal Surgery, Royal Orthopaedic Hospital, Birmingham

Roger Tillman FRCS(Orth), Consultant Orthopaedic Oncologist, Royal Orthopaedic Hospital Birmingham and Chairman, British Orthopaedic Association Committee for Best Practice in the Management of Bone Disease, London

David A Tolley MD FRCS FRCS(Ed), Director and Consultant Urologist, Scottish Lithotriptor Centre, Western General Hospital, Edinburgh

Paul A Vasey MD MSc FRCP, Senior Lecturer in Medical Oncology, Beatson Oncology Centre, Glasgow

D Mike A Wallace FRCS, Consultant Urological Surgeon, Queen Elizabeth Hospital, Birmingham

David C Wilson MB BS MRCP FRCR, Specialist Registrar in Clinical Oncology, CRC Institute for Cancer Studies, University of Birmingham, Birmingham

Annie Young RGN BSc MSc, Honorary Research Fellow, Cancer Research UK Institute for Cancer Studies, University of Birmingham, Birmingham

Preface

Kidney cancer, the majority of which is renal cell carcinoma (RCC), accounts for about 2% of all cancers world-wide, although the incidence rates vary over three-fold, with the highest rates in Northern Europe and the lowest rates in Asia. The incidence of RCC has been increasing in many populations, partly due to the increased detection of asymptomatic tumours. However, mortality rates have also increased in most Western populations, suggesting that exposure to environmental risk factors associated with an affluent lifestyle are important in the development of this disease. In Chapter One, Allen provides a particularly thorough review of the epidemiology of RCC, discussing the genetic, environmental and medical risk factors that have been implicated in the genesis of the disease. Established risk factors, she notes, include a family history of RCC, previous kidney disease or injury, cigarette smoking and obesity.

Genetic factors are seen to account for a very small proportion of cases while in contrast environmental factors such as smoking and obesity may together combine to account for up to 30% of RCC in men and 40% in women. The role of other factors in the aetiology of RCC is less clear although suspected medical risk factors include hypertension and/or its treatment, and prolonged use of analgesics. The evidence that RCC is associated with diet, particularly with a high red meat intake and a low fruit and vegetable intake, is inconsistent as is the evidence that occupational exposure to asbestos, coke oven emissions, petrol and solvents are associated with RCC, but it certainly appears sensible that current efforts to reduce the increasing trend of RCC in many Western populations should focus on reducing the prevalence of smoking and give attention to the dietary risk factors that have been implicated in research studies to date.

In Chapter Two, Maher is concerned to examine the molecular and clinical genetics of RCC with particular reference to how our current knowledge may help in the identification of the individual at risk of disease. Inherited renal tumours are infrequent, as Maher points out, but nevertheless important because of the opportunities for reducing morbidity and mortality by targeted screening. In a fascinating overview the author describes the relative importance and characteristics of the genetic basis of renal cell cancers, including study of familial renal cell carcinoma (RCC), a genetically heterogeneous disease and clear cell RCC with its relationship to the dominantly inherited multisystem cancer syndrome that is von Hippel-Lindau (VHL) disease. Of particular interest in this context is the identification of the VHL gene which has enabled the provision of reliable genetic testing to be offered to VHL families and thus a significantly enhanced management of susceptibility. In addition to this particular category of disease, Maher describes a group of patients with familial non-VHL clear cell RCC but for whom there is at present no genetic tests available for kindreds.

A further variant, familial papillary (non-clear cell) RCC may, as the author describes, result from germline mutations in the MET proto-oncogene and tumours from these patients typically show type 1 papillary RCC where the detection of germline MET gene mutations allows accurate genetic diagnosis of at risk relatives within affected families. More rarely, RCC may be associated with tuberous sclerosis, but angiomyolipomas are the major renal tumour in this disorder. Recently, an association between non-clear cell RCC and Birt-Hogg-Dube (BHD) syndrome has been reported, the latter condition being characterised by the association of cutaneous fibrofolliculomas with lipomas and spontaneous pneumothorax. These developments in our understanding of the molecular genetics of RCC are of considerable importance because, as Maher is clear, an early recognition of individuals at high risk of RCC enables these particular patients to be afforded access to techniques such as annual renal ultrasound surveillance, which can directly reduce morbidity and mortality from the disease, while low risk relatives can be properly reassured.

We move from the overview of epidemiology in Chapter One and molecular and clinical genetics in Chapter Two to a detailed exposition of current thinking on the natural history of renal call cancer in Chapter Three. The natural history of untreated disease is to invade locally, infiltrate into the venous circulation and to metastasise to lymph nodes and distant organs, especially the lung, with variable rates of progression. As Oliver describes, it is now more than 30 years since Everson and Cole reviewed the occurrence of spontaneous regression of cancer in the world literature, being the first investigators to highlight the fact that renal cell cancer had nearly the highest frequency of such an event. Oliver describes his own personal interest in RCC as extending back over some twenty four years, beginning with the experience of his first renal cancer patient treated with chemotherapy. The patient had lived with a solitary, slow growing lung metatasis for nearly ten years which was beginning to become symptomatic. Three weeks after a single dose of cyclophosphamide the patient developed widespread multiple lung metastases and was dead within six weeks. At that time there was considerable controversy regarding the frequency with which spontaneous regression of RCC occurred with one prominent author calculating an estimate of 0.3% from a literature based study while another observed a rate of 30% non-progression at six months in a personal series of 35 untreated metastatic renal cancer patients.

This polarity of view and the increasing recognition of the impact of patient selection on outcome of treatment led Oliver to conduct a prospective study of disease frequency in the setting of the good performance status patients referred to tertiary centres which undertake clinical trials. An increasingly recognized characteristic of trials in renal cell cancer was that initial reports were often double that achieved when the treatment became generally available. Because of this, Oliver describes how he considered it vital to exclude the possibility that the responses reported for biological treatment simply reflected episodes of spontaneous regression in the highly selected subgroup referred to these specialist centres. In order to investigate this further, the author describes how patients with early but symptomatic metastases underwent a period of surveillance to investigate what was the frequency of spontaneous regression and to investigate whether there was any relation between spontaneous regression and response to cytokine therapy.

Oliver describes how an initial report of the first seventy two patients observed a 7% spontaneous regression rate and an additional 7% non-progression rate at 12 months and goes on to update the results from this study to report a total of 292 of patients entered. Examination of the results has shown that while the response rate has fallen to 4%, the response continues to be durable. Usefully, the chapter reviews possible factors involved in the effect of this study on response in subsequent cytokine studies and discusses how these new observations may be relevant for increasing interest in the use of cytokines as a pre-operative treatment for renal cell patients prior to surgery and how they might have a more generalised application in the therapy of all primary cancers.

Part Two of the volume is concerned to examine the role of histopathology and imaging in the diagnosis and staging of renal cell carcinoma. In Chapter Four, Howie describes precisely how pathologists contribute to the management of RCC by posing and answering three specific questions. Firstly, is the diagnosis renal cell carcinoma rather than something else? Secondly, what type of renal cell carcinoma is it? Thirdly, what features are present of relevance to prognosis? The importance of these specific though hardly simple questions is clearly seen throughout the chapter. Indeed, there are supposedly benign neoplasms of the kidney that may be confused with renal cell carcinoma, namely papillary adenoma, metanephric adenoma and oncocytoma.

The author reminds us that the current classification of renal cell carcinoma is into common or conventional clear cell carcinoma, two types of papillary carcinoma, chromophobe carcinoma, collecting duct carcinoma and unclassified carcinoma. Sarcomatoid change is seen in all types and is widely recognised as an indicator of poor prognosis. The most important prognostic feature in renal cell carcinoma is, as with many tumour types, the extent of spread and it is in this context that the pathologist ideally provides information from which the stage can be determined by someone who is aware of all of the relevant facts. In the TNM system, stage one corresponds with T1, that is, a carcinoma no more than 7 cm diameter without spread into major veins or outside the kidney. Stage two corresponds with T2, a carcinoma over 7 cm diameter, but otherwise similar to stage one. Stage three means spread into veins, T3b or T3c, and/or into the adrenal gland or perinephric fat, T3a, and/or into one lymph node, N1. Stage four means spread into adjacent organs other than adrenal gland, T4, and/or into more than one lymph node, N2, and/or into a distant organ, M1.

The review of the central role of histopathology services provided by Howie is entirely complemented in Chapter Five by Kabala in his detailed description of the place of diagnostic imaging in renal cancer. As he points out, the initial radiological investigation of haematuria remains controversial and in recent years it has been increasingly argued that ultrasound can displace IVU. The advantages are, certainly, the avoidance of radiation and intravenous contrast and the availability and speed of the procedure itself but Kabala is clear that while ultrasound is more sensitive than IVU for the detection of masses it is highly likely to miss small upper tract urothelial malignancies and occasionally RCC. These observations have led to the suggestion that both ultrasound and IVU should therefore logically be performed but even in macroscopic haematuria over 50% of patients will have no diagnosis made and the IVU will therefore be redundant. The author argues that in the very few patients in whom a small urothelial tumour is not shown on ultrasound, further investigation has the strong potential to detect the lesion prior to its significant progression by, for example, arranging IVU if the patient has recurrent or persistent haematuria.

Following detection of a mass, ultrasound will categorise it as a simple cyst (in the vast majority of cases) or as a malignant renal mass in at least 90% of cases with approximately 80–85 % of solid masses representing renal cell carcinoma. The remaining renal masses are to some extent indeterminate; being neither an obvious benign cyst nor an obvious RCC. The author is clear that all of these require further investigation with CT or MRI and can be classified into four categories ranging from simple cysts to tumours with substantial enhancing solid areas. Approximately 90% of category IV lesions and 60% of category III lesions are malignant and justify surgery with approximately 25–30% of category II lesions being malignant. Image guided aspiration of cyst fluid for cytology and interval scanning if no malignant cells are found is likely to be safe for these lesions.

The author goes on to illustrate how both CT and MRI can stage RCC with similar high accuracy except in the distinction of totally confined renal cell carcinoma from tumours that have extended through the capsule. The error rate for this is of the order of 50%. This is of little importance in radical nephrectomy but becomes more significant where nephron sparing surgery (partial nephrectomy) is considered. Partial nephrectomy also depends on being able to preserve a separate blood supply to the remaining healthy renal tissue and therefore generally requires pre-operative assessment of the renal vasculature which can be reliably performed with MR or CT angiography.

We have dedicated Part Three of this volume to a detailed consideration of the current evidence base for surgical intervention in the management of renal cell carcinoma. At the time of writing there are no meta-analyses and few randomised trials to guide the management of localised renal cell carcinoma and it is true to say that what evidence there is to support treatment derives largely from observational studies relating the surgical and pathological extent of disease to survival with the interpretation of the data on survival over time being obscured by changes in disease staging systems, as Richards and Ritchie point out. Five year survival of 3% has been reported for 'operable' patients having no treatment and the 'received wisdom', which has as its basis the conventional approach of nephrectomy with as wide a margin of normal tissue as possible, has increasingly been challenged by improved pre-operative imaging procedures and the experience gained from less radical intervention for small tumours.

Historical evidence suggests that simple nephrectomy improves survival over conservative management. Simple nephrectomy results in poor 5-year survival rates for stage II disease but the advantages of radical over simple nephrectomy remain controversial. The pattern of lymph node spread is not predictable and while some retrospective studies suggest that lymphadenectomy improves survival in Robson stage II and III disease, and while it is generally agreed that that lymphadenectomy combined with radical nephrectomy does not increase morbidity or mortality, there are no reliable studies within the literature to date which have been able confidently to report on survival benefits. Categorisation of vena caval extension into four levels has helped to minimise morbidity but management of level 3 extension remains controversial. Five year survival of 64% can be achieved even if the disease extends to the atrium and the introduction of new surgical techniques is an opportunity to undertake prospective randomised studies which in turn can be expected to provide better evidence.

Nephron sparing surgery, the subject of Chapter Seven, is a complex surgical technique with an appreciable learning curve. It remains indicated in patients with a tumour in a solitary kidney and accumulating surgical experience together with the evolution and refinement of the technique has led some authorities to advocate this particular surgical intervention in patients with small tumours with a normal contralateral kidney. Nephron sparing surgery in this context, as Aitchison and Bromwich describe, provides a safe and comparable oncological outcome to the standard treatment of radical nephrectomy but the authors are clear that the evidence for this is based on comparative single institution studies and no randomised controlled clinical trial comparing nephron sparing surgery with radical nephrectomy has yet been completed. New techniques and technologies may come to provide an alternative to open partial nephrectomy with a better outcome but these will require careful evaluation in significant numbers of patients and an adequate length of follow up.

Laparoscopic surgical approaches to the management of renal cancer, for example, remain of much interest but in order to become established as an acceptable alternative treatment for surgically resectable renal cell carcinoma, the laparoscopic approach must fulfil certain criteria. Jones and Tolley, writing in Chapter Eight, enumerate two of these that they consider central to the utility of the technique: the surgical outcome must be equivalent or better than incisional surgery and the oncological outcome must be at least equivalent. In terms of the evidence available to address these concerns, the authors cite a meta-analysis of the relevant literature which demonstrates that laparoscopic nephrectomy for benign disease results in a shorter hospital stay, lower rate of blood transfusion and fewer complications. These benefits, which are impressive in nature, are similarly seen in patients undergoing laparoscopic radical nephrectomy for malignant disease.

Laparoscopic radical nephrectomy, as Jones and Tolley describe, was first performed in 1991 and since that time experience in the use of the technique has been essentially limited, being restricted to a relatively small number of international centres. Experience with laparoscopic partial nephrectomy is similarly limited with an oncological outcome comparable to that reported for incisional partial nephrectomy. These authors conclude that these techniques may therefore be regarded as in many ways superior in surgical outcome to incisional surgery and should be offered as the first choice procedure to patients with T1 lesions who would otherwise undergo conventional radical surgery.

Part Four of this volume is focused on the current evidence base for medical intervention in the management of renal cell carcinoma. In the first chapter of this section, Hess and Gore contribute a stimulating review of the place of cytokine treatment in rencal cell cancer. As the authors note, while RCC rarely responds to chemotherapy or hormone therapy, it is well recognised that the tumour responds well to immunotherapy and there is now a large literature on the use of cytokines for the treatment of this disease. Interferon alpha results in response rates of about 15% but complete remissions are rare and are typically in the region of 2%. Experience its use has led to general agreement on the dosing schedules that appear most appropriate but not on the optimal duration of therapy which remains a matter of controversy. Typically, as the authors describe, patients are assessed every 3 months and provided that there is a tumour response or a stabilization of disease, treatment is continued if side effects are tolerable. This is because late responses after 6–12 months of treatment are recorded. It is not known, as they point out, whether there is any benefit for continuing interferon therapy over one year in a patient who has responded.

Single agent interleukin-2 (IL-2) results in similar response rates to interferon alpha although the data suggest that complete remission may occur slightly more frequently (5–10%). Long term complete remissions are, certainly, recorded, but only in regimens using IV boluses of high dose IL-2, which is a rather toxic schedule. Furthermore, these data have not been confirmed in randomised trials. There appears, as Hess and Gore discuss, to be no advantage to combining interferon alpha or LAK cells with IL-2 but there has been great interest over the last ten years of combining interferon alpha, IL-2 and 5-FU, with response rates of 40% being reported. Unfortunately, however, what data there are are inconsistent and even the 2 randomised trials assessing this combination report very different results with these inconsistencies perhaps due to differences in the scheduling of the cytokines or patient selection between the studies.

Randomised trials and a Cochrane review demonstrate that interferon alpha therapy is associated with a survival benefit for patients with metastatic disease and this is the standard care for fit patients. Patients who are unfit, particularly if they have multiple sites of disease and rapidly progressing tumours, do not benefit from cytokine therapy. Studies comparing interferon alpha with interferon alpha plus IL-2 plus 5-FU in fit patients with metastatic disease have been conducted and the analysis and interpretation of their results is awaited with much interest.

Certain patients with non-metastatic disease are candidates for adjuvant therapy trials. Important risk factors for relapse in pT3 tumours include the presence of extrarenal invasion, positive surgical margins and renal hilar lymphadenopathy. Possible options for adjuvant strategies include hormones, chemotherapy, radiotherapy and immunotherapy and it is to a consideration of the relative merits of these options that O'Neill and Vasey turn in Chapter Ten. Hormones such as medroxyprogesterone and conventional cytotoxics are not significantly active in RCC, and are not suitable for adjuvant therapy. The main criteria for a successful adjuvant approach is the ability to predict a higher risk of relapse based on tumour-specific features and the availability of an active regimen. Radiotherapy is an effective treatment in the palliative setting but retains a debatable role in primary therapy. As an adjunct to surgery, it has been associated with improved survival rates in retrospective studies but not in prospective randomised trials. Further studies are necessary definitively to outline any benefit, but as most patients relapse with distant metastases and not local recurrences, radiotherapy may not be the most effective adjuvant treatment. Immunotherapy with interferon-alpha has demonstrated improved survival over hormonal therapy in randomised studies and interleukin-2 (IL-2) has been shown to be associated with durable clinical responses in metastatic disease. Combinations of IFA and IL-2 are associated with more toxicity and higher response rates than each individual cytokine and combination with 5-fluorouracil may well show response rates in excess of 30%.

Responses to biotherapy or bio-chemotherapy have been modest at the expense of profound systemic toxicity, as Pandha and colleagues point out in Chapter Eleven. This has led, as they discuss, to the development of novel approaches for treatment and three specific strategies based on manipulation of the immune system are currently being investigated. Thalidomide, for example, has been shown to be clinically useful in a number of inflammatory disorders and cancers including renal cell cancer. The activity of this agent has been attributed to its wide ranging immunological and non-immunological effects including anti-TNF-alpha activity, T cell co-stimulation, anti-angiogenic activities and also direct anti-tumour activity. The design of compounds based on thalidomide structure has led to the synthesis of analogues with enhanced selectivity, immunological activity and reduced toxicity to humans and these agents, currently under investigation, are most conveniently categorised as selective cytokine inhibitory drugs (SelCIDs) and immunomodulatory drugs (IMiDs).

Dendritic cells are potent antigen-presenting cells involved in the initiation of antigen-specific immune responses and are the basis of the second novel approach to therapy which Pandha and his colleagues describe. The ability to generate and cryopreserve large numbers of these cells *in vitro* has, as they show, facilitated a number of cancer vaccine strategies and further manipulation of these cells by pulsing, transfecting or fusing with tumour antigen or tumour cells has shown them capable of generating significant clinical responses in renal cell cancer patients. A third novel approach to therapy discussed by the authors is represented by allogeneic bone marrow transplantation which is well recognised to induce powerful graft-versus-leukaemia effects in patients with haematological malignancies providing evidence of a graft-versus tumour effect in patients with solid tumours. A relatively recent approach to the use of this therapy in renal cell cancer has involved, as Pandha and associates outline, the use of non-myeloablative chemotherapy to suppress the immune system sufficiently to engraft allogeneic peripheral blood stem cells in patients with metastatic renal cell carcinoma. Initial studies have demonstrated that sustained regression of tumour is possible in patients unresponsive to conventional treatment with acceptable toxicity and the results of further study of this intervention are awaited with interest.

The final chapter in Part Four of this text, Chapter Twelve, provides an overview of the prognostic factors that are considered to be of direct relevance to the management of renal cell carcinoma. James and Wilson make the point that the disease has an extremely variable prognosis and that stage alone does not adequately describe the full range of prognostic possibilities. As there is growing evidence that certain treatments for relapsed or metastatic disease may improve survival, the authors believe it increasingly important to formulate a prognosis accurately to allow effective case selection. This is particularly true as palliative options now include nephrectomy (improvement in median survival of around 50%) and immunotherapy with interferon (improvement in median survival of around 28%). The authors emphasise that in order for patients to derive worthwhile benefit from interventions such as nephrectomy, it is essential that they have a reasonable estimated survival in the first place. In this context, a number of factors need to be considered in assessing prognosis and, for James and Wilson, the principal elements are pathology, performance status, stage and choice of treatment.

We have dedicated Part Five of this volume, the penultimate part, to current thinking on the management of metastases from renal cell cancers which seed to the spine, to the pelvis and to the extremities. Bone metastases occur in approximately 60% of patients with renal carcinoma. Historically, the outcome from spinal metastatic disease has been poor and the results of early surgical studies have shown that the largely inappropriate and inadequate techniques adopted resulted in outcomes that were no better than conventional radiotherapy and steroids.

The usual manifestations of spinal metastases are, of course, intractable pain due to mechanical instability secondary to pathological fracture with or without neurological compromise. Dramatic improvements in orthopaedic spinal surgery, as Stirling and his associates discuss, now permit a graduated surgical response proportionate to the individual's prognosis and the exact nature of the spinal pathology.

These include techniques of extra-lesional, intra-lesional (or marginal) resection and reconstruction or palliation with decompression and stabilisation. If, on the basis of tumour characterisation and staging, patients with a good prognosis can be identified, more aggressive surgical techniques should be considered with radiotherapy being reserved for those patients not well enough for, or amenable to, techniques of resection or palliative stabilisation. Preoperative embolisation is recommended providing significantly reduced blood loss and facilitation of the operation.

Appropriate management of bone metastases is therefore, as Patton and his colleagues go on to discuss in Chapter Fourteen in their review of the management of metastases to the appendicular skeleton, essential in order to prevent the morbidity associated with pathological fractures and failed fixation devices, to optimise the function of the patient and to minimise the associated pain. Factors that should be taken into consideration when dealing with bone metastases and guidelines for when orthopaedic intervention may be required are discussed. As is so often the case, the importance of good communication across specialities is emphasised.

Part Six of this volume, the final part, opens and concludes with a consideration of two issues of central concern to the good clinical governance of renal cancer services: clinical audit and the provision of information as part of shared decision making between clinician and patient. Clinical audit, for example, as James and Wallace discuss, is a key component of modern medical practice and of central importance for both clinical governance and quality assurance. Acknowledging that national comparative data are hard to obtain in a timely fashion and suffer from variations in methodology, time lags in collection, inconsistency of coding and logistic constraints on data entry and analysis, the authors present and discuss a novel web-based tool for online national audit which they advance as being of no small value to the development of the quality of clinical practice in the management of renal cell carcinoma. In illustration of the potential of this technique, the authors present selected data generated by an audit of head and neck cancer carried out under the auspices of the Audit Committee of The Royal College of Radiologists.

In modern clinical practice patients increasingly seek and demand the information which will enable them to achieve a greater understanding of their disease or condition. In the final chapter of this volume, Daniels and associates report their initial findings from a study of the acceptability and usefulness of the world wide web as a cancer information resource and discuss how their findings may prove relevant for the provision of information in this manner to patients with renal cell cancer.

In the current age, where doctors and health professionals are increasingly overwhelmed by clinical information, we have aimed to provide a fully current, fully referenced text which is as succinct as possible but as comprehensive as necessary. Consultants in Urology, Medical and Clinical Oncology and their trainees are likely to find it of particular use as part of continuing professional development and specialist training respectively and we advance it specifically as an excellent tool for this purpose. We anticipate that the book will, in addition, prove invaluable to clinical nurse specialists in urology and oncology and to oncology pharmacists and to the commissioners and planners of cancer services when in dialogue with their specialist colleagues.

In conclusion, we thank Roche Products Ltd and Chiron Ltd for the grant of unconditional educational sponsorship which helped organise a national symposium on renal cell cancer held with the British Association of Urological Surgeons, The Royal College of Radiologists and the Association of Cancer Physicians at The Royal College of Pathologists at which synopses of the individual chapters of this book were presented. Our thanks are also due to Kidney Cancer UK for their interest in and attendance at the national meeting.

Michael Aitchison MD FRCS
Tim Oliver MD FRCP
Andrew Miles MSc MPhil PhD

Acknowledgements

The following colleagues contributed as members of the expert planning committee for the RCC project: Mr. Michael Aitchison, Professor Martin Gore, Professor Nicholas James, Professor Andrew Miles, Professor Tim Oliver, Mr. Alastair Ritchie, Mr. Alistair Stirling, Mr. Michael Wallace. The contribution of Dr. Andreas Polychronis, Research Fellow/Specialist Registrar in Medical Oncology, Imperial College at the Hammersmith Hospital London as Secretary to the Committee and Assistant Editor in the preparation of the current volume, is also acknowledged.

PART 1

Epidemiology, genetics and risk

Chapter 1

The epidemiology of renal cell carcinoma: rates and risk factors

Naomi E Allen

Kidney cancer accounts for approximately 4800 cancer cases and 2700 deaths each year in England and Wales (Office for National Statistics 2001). With the ageing of the population and the gradual rise in kidney cancer incidence and mortality rates over recent years, this disease is set to become an increasing public health burden. This chapter aims to give a description of the geographical and temporal trends in kidney cancer incidence and mortality, with a focus on renal cell carcinoma (RCC), the predominant form of kidney cancer. An outline of the risk factors involved in the aetiology of the disease is then provided, with an emphasis on environmental risk factors and the potential for future cancer prevention.

Incidence and mortality rates

It is estimated that there are about 95 000–100 000 new cases of kidney cancer worldwide each year, accounting for about 1.5% of all cancers diagnosed and 2% of all cancer deaths. In England and Wales, kidney cancer was diagnosed in about 3000 men and 1800 women in 1997 alone, making it the eighth most common cancer in men and the fourteenth most common cancer in women (Office for National Statistics 2001).

About 80–90% of the malignant tumours in both sexes occur in the kidney parenchyma (renal cortex), 5–10% occur in the renal pelvis and 5% in the ureter. Wilms' tumour, or nephroblastoma, is the most common childhood cancer of the kidney and accounts for approximately 2% of all kidney cases. The majority of renal cell cancers are adenocarcinomas, arising from the renal tubular cells; in contrast, most cancers of the renal pelvis and ureter are transitional cell carcinomas and are therefore anatomically and histologically distinct from RCC.

A relatively high percentage of patients (25–30%) present with metastases at clinical diagnosis, the most common sites being the lung, bone and liver, although any organ can be affected (Motzer et al. 1996). The mortality rate for kidney cancer is therefore relatively high, and up to 50% of patients do not survive longer than 5 years after initial diagnosis. In 1997, there were about 1600 deaths from kidney cancer in men and 1000 deaths in women in England and Wales alone, making the prognosis of kidney cancer worse than that for prostate or bladder cancer, the other main cancers of the urogenital tract (Office for National Statistics 2001). Kidney cancer now accounts for more deaths each year than cancer of the brain, oral cavity and liver, and malignant melanoma of the skin.

Over the age of 35 years, the incidence and mortality rates for men are consistently higher than for women, with rate ratios generally between 1.5:1 and 2.5:1. In both sexes, the incidence rates increase with age and over 45% of cases occur in those aged 65–79 years (Office for National Statistics 2001) (Figure 1.1).

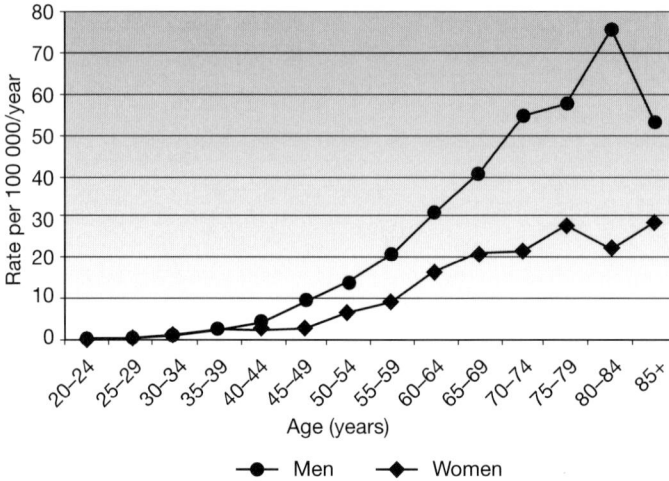

Figure 1.1 Age-specific incidence rates of kidney cancer in England and Wales, 1997. Data are taken from the Office for National Statistics (2001).

Geographical trends

Historically, incidence rates for kidney cancer have included RCC together with tumours of the renal pelvis and ureter, despite their different characteristics. There are limited data on the rates of RCC alone and, as rates for kidney cancer as a whole largely reflect those of RCC, the incidence and mortality rates are presented here for all kidney cancers.

There is an approximate sixfold variation in the incidence of kidney cancer around the world. Generally, the highest rates occur in northern and western Europe, North America and Australia where there are about 11–13 cases diagnosed per 100 000 men per year and about 4–7 cases per 100 000 women per year. The lowest rates are in Asia and Africa, and are generally less than 6/100 000 per year in men and less than 3/100 000 per year in women (Ferlay et al. 2001). Kidney cancer rates in the UK are intermediate and are approximately 8/100 000 per year in men and 4/100 000 per year in women, when age-standardised to the world population (Figure 1.2). Differences in kidney cancer rates also exist within a country and have been reported to be higher among black Americans than in white Americans in both men and women (Chow et al. 1999).

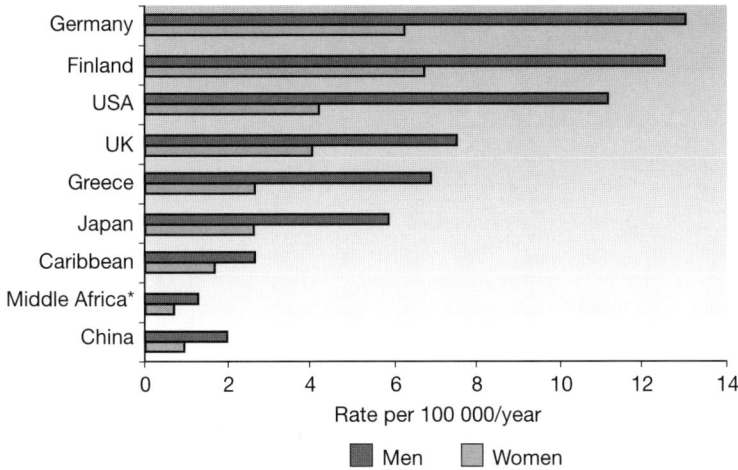

Figure 1.2 Estimated international kidney cancer incidence rates in selected countries for the year 2000. Rates are standardised to the world population. Data are taken from the Globocan 2000 Database (Ferlay et al. 2001).

*Rates are an average for Angola, Cameroon, Central African Republic, Chad, Congo Brazzaville, Congo, Equatorial Guinea and Gabon.

Mortality rates follow the same pattern as incidence rates, with the highest rates observed in northern and western European countries, being between 4 and 8/100 000 per year in men and 2 and 3/100 000 per year in women. The lowest rates are observed in Asia and Africa and are generally less than 3/100 000 per year in men and 1.5/100 000 per year in women (Figure 1.3). Again, figures for the UK are intermediate, being 4/100 000 per year in men and 2/100 000 per year in women (World Health Organization 2001). Evidence from migrant studies is limited, although one study reported an increase in kidney cancer mortality among south Europeans 30 years after moving to Australia (McCredie et al. 1999). This observation, together with the wide variation in cancer mortality rates between countries, suggests that environmental as well as genetic factors may be important in the aetiology of this disease. Kidney cancer incidence and mortality tend to be higher in urban compared with rural populations, especially among men, but there is no consistent association with education or socioeconomic status across populations (McLaughlin et al. 1996). However, the pattern of risk between countries suggests that this cancer is associated with a Western lifestyle.

Temporal trends

The incidence of kidney cancer has been increasing in nearly every country, but particularly in North America and northern Europe (Ries et al. 2001) (Figure 1.4).

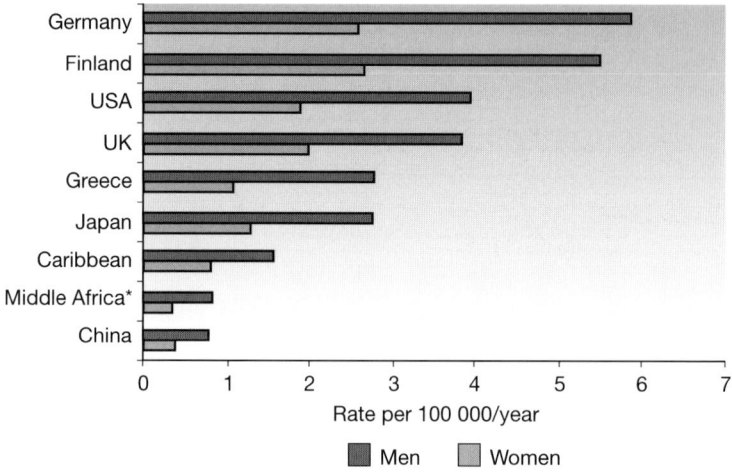

Figure 1.3 Estimated international kidney cancer mortality rates in selected countries for the year 2000. Rates are standardised to the world population. Data taken from the WHO Mortality Databank (2001).
*Rates are an average for Angola, Cameroon, Central African Republic, Chad, Congo Brazzaville, Congo, Equatorial Guinea and Gabon.

Indeed, over the last 30 years, kidney cancer incidence in Western countries has increased at a faster rate than any other common cancer other than non-Hodgkin's lymphoma, melanoma, prostate cancer in men and lung cancer in women. In the UK, age-adjusted incidence rates have doubled from 5.5 to 12/100 000 per year in men and from 3.4 to 6.8/100 000 per year in women between 1971 and 1997 (Figure 1.4). This increase over time is apparent in all age groups, but particularly between the ages of 65 and 74 years. This is mostly the result of increased detection of small and non-symptomatic tumours, which are found incidentally during clinical investigations for other kidney conditions (Smith et al. 1989). Indeed, there is evidence to suggest that between 25% and 40% of kidney tumours are detected after the use of imaging procedures such as abdominal ultrasonography, computed tomography and magnetic resonance imaging (Motzer et al. 1996). However, a study in the USA suggests that the use of diagnostic tools does not explain all of the rise in incidence observed in this country, because the incidence of high-stage, metastatic tumours has also increased over time (Chow et al. 1999).

Further, kidney cancer mortality rates have also steadily increased over the last 30 years in both sexes. This is in contrast to most other cancers, such as cancer of the lung, stomach, bladder and colorectum, the mortality rates of which have been gradually declining, in recent years (Figure 1.5). The steady increase in kidney cancer mortality over the last 30 years has occurred in most populations, with the

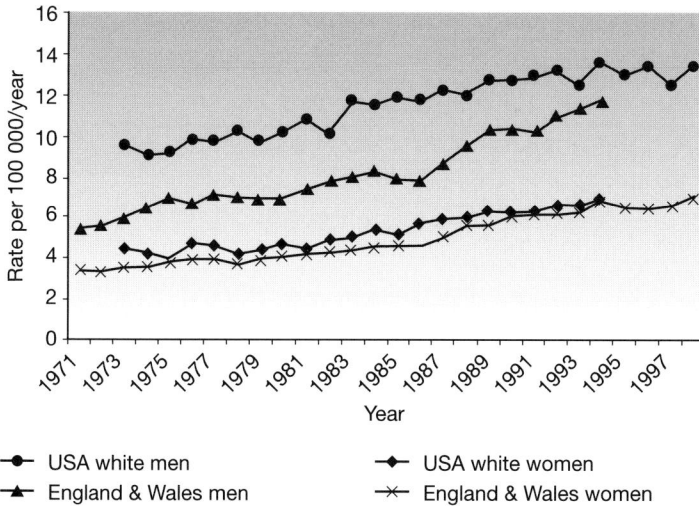

Figure 1.4 Kidney cancer incidence rates in the USA and England and Wales, 1971–1998. Rates are adjusted to the national populations. Data for England and Wales are taken from the Office for National Statistics (2001). Data for the USA are taken from the SEER Cancer Statistical Review, 1973–1998 (Ries et al. 2001).

largest increases in men being observed in Japan and among black Americans, rising by 140% and 68%, respectively (Figure 1.6). Mortality rates have increased by a lesser extent among British and white American men, but nevertheless have risen by 34% and 16%, respectively (Ries et al. 2001; WHO 2001) (Figure 1.6). The increase in mortality rates over time in low- and high-incidence countries shows a similar pattern among women, with the largest increases observed in Japan and among black American women (Figure 1.7). These observations strongly suggest that increased exposure to some environmental risk factor(s), perhaps associated with the adoption of a Western-type lifestyle, is important in the development of the disease.

Trends in survival

The prognosis of patients diagnosed with kidney cancer has generally improved over time, as a result of earlier detection and subsequent treatment of localised, often incidental, tumours. Five-year survival rates among white people in the USA increased from about 50% during the period 1975–85 to 60% during the period 1986–95; however, 5-year survival rates have not improved as much for black Americans and were reported to be 50% for men and 58% for women during the period 1986–95 (Chow et al. 1999). Survival rates tend to be lower in Europe, and were estimated to be between 48% and 50% during the period 1985–89 (Damhuis and Kirkels 1998).

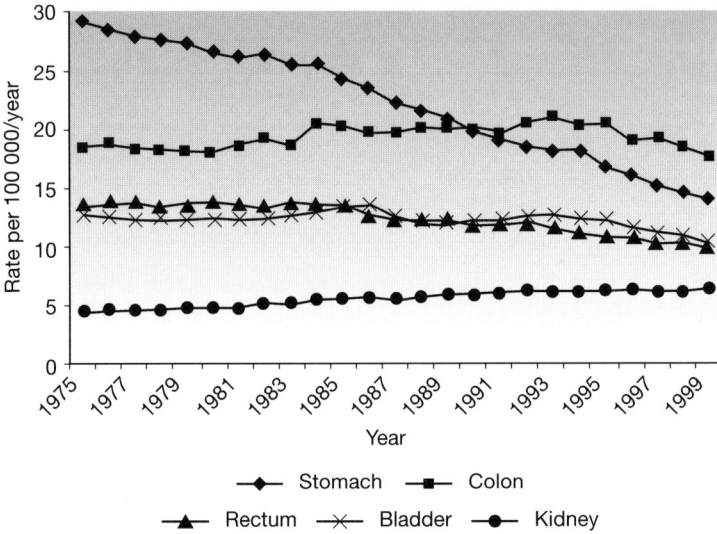

Figure 1.5 Cancer mortality rates in men, England and Wales 1975–1999. Rates are standardised to the England and Wales population. Data are taken from the Office for National Statistics (2001).

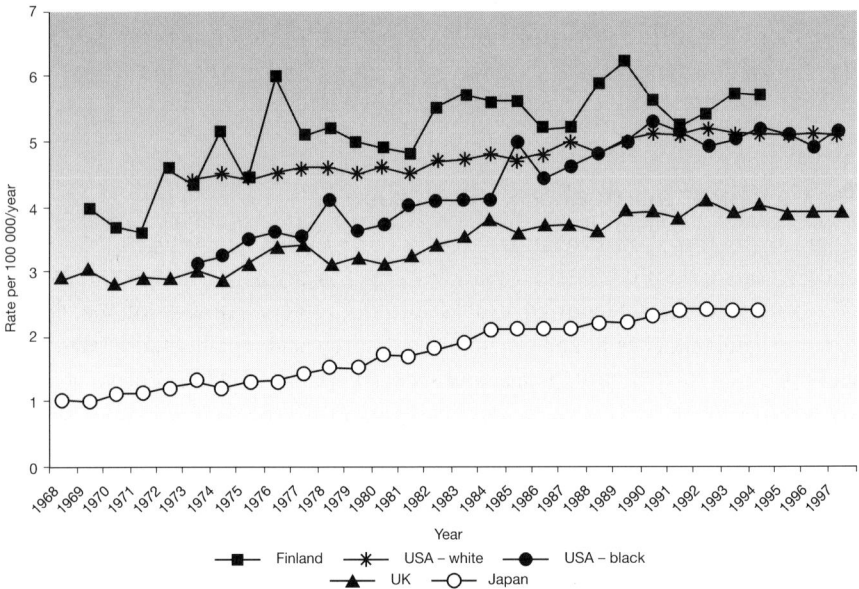

Figure 1.6 Kidney cancer mortality rates in men for selected countries 1969–1997. Rates are standarised to the world population, except the USA (standardised to 1970 US population). Data for Finland, UK and Japan are taken from the WHO Mortality Database (2001). Data for the USA taken from the Seer Cancer Statistics Review, 1973–1998 (Ries et al. 2001).

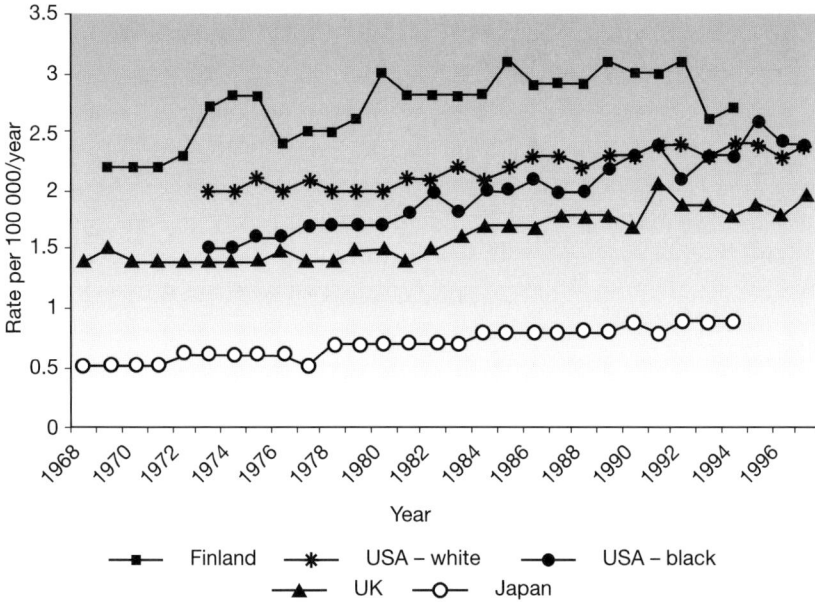

Figure 1.7 Kidney cancer mortality rates in women for selected countries 1969–1997. Rates are standarised to the world population, except the USA (standardised to 1970 US population). Data for Finland, UK and Japan are taken from the WHO Mortality Database (2001). Data for the USA taken from the Seer Cancer Statistics Review, 1973–1998 (Ries et al. 2001).

Risk factors for renal cell carcinoma

Relatively little is known about the aetiology of RCC, which has been the focus of epidemiological research only in the last few years, largely in the form of observational case–control studies. Identified causes include a family history of the disease, cigarette smoking, obesity and previous renal injury, and together these factors may account for up to 40% of RCC cases in men and women. Little is known about the influence of other factors, although the pattern of risk between countries suggests that this cancer is associated with an affluent lifestyle. Suspected risk factors include hypertension and/or its medications, the use of analgesics, diet and occupational factors, but the evidence is inconsistent and probably accounts for a smaller proportion of cases.

Established risk factors

Hereditary renal cell carcinoma

There are believed to be three inherited forms of RCC, all of which are rare and dominantly inherited, and which account for a small, but unknown, proportion of cases. Having a first-degree family member with a diagnosis of RCC, especially at a young age (30–50 years) increases the risk of hereditary renal cell carcinoma by about twofold (Schlehofer et al. 1996) and has been associated with a germ-line mutation on the short arm of chromosome 3 (3p) (Latif et al. 1993). Secondly, 25–45% of individuals with von Hippel–Lindau (VHL) syndrome, a rare inherited autosomal dominant cancer syndrome, go on to develop clear-cell renal adenocarcinomas (Lamiell et al. 1989; Neumann et al. 1995), as well as cancers at other sites. A third hereditary form is papillary RCC, which is histologically and genetically distinct from VHL disease, being characterised by multifocal papillary tumours, which are linked to inherited genetic mutations in the *Met* proto-oncogene on the long arm of chromosome 7 (7q) (Schmidt et al. 1997).

Deletions of 3p and associated allele losses have been reported in up to 75% of sporadic renal carcinomas (Gnarra 1998) and somatic mutations of the *Met* gene have also been described in some sporadic cases of papillary tumours of the kidney (Schmidt et al. 1997). This strongly suggests that sporadic and hereditary RCC may arise through common genetic mechanisms. However, as most RCCs are sporadic, the genetic changes involved in kidney tumorigenesis are not inherited and occur after birth, possibly as a result of exposure to environmental risk factors such as cigarette smoke, occupational hazards and dietary factors.

Cigarette smoking

The most long-established environmental risk factor identified with RCC is cigarette smoking. Evidence from case–control and cohort studies have shown smokers to have a twofold increased risk of developing RCC compared with non-smokers in both men and women (McLaughlin et al. 1984, 1990, 1992a; Maclure and Willett 1990; McCredie and Stewart 1992b; Kreiger et al. 1993; Yuan et al. 1998b; Chow et al. 2000). It has been estimated that cigarette smoking may account for 20–30% of cases of RCC in men and 10–20% in women (McLaughlin et al. 1995b; Yuan et al. 1998b). There is also strong evidence for a dose–response relationship between duration and frequency of cigarette smoking and RCC risk (McLaughlin et al. 1984, 1995b; Maclure and Willett 1990; Kreiger et al. 1993; Yuan et al. 1998b), whereas smoking cessation results in a 15–30% reduction in risk after 10–15 years (McLaughlin et al. 1995b; Yuan et al. 1998b). Cigar smoking has also been associated with an increased risk of RCC, independent of cigarette smoking (Yuan et al. 1998b), although other studies have not found any association (Yu et al. 1986; McLaughlin et al. 1995b). It has been suggested that carcinogens in tobacco smoke, such as *N*-nitrosodimethylamine, which has been shown to cause kidney tumours in animals (IARC 1986), may become concentrated in the kidney and damage kidney cell DNA, although the precise mechanism is not known. However, the level of increased risk of RCC with smoking is well below that observed with cancer of the renal pelvis and ureter (McCredie et al. 1983a; Ross et al. 1989; McLaughlin et al. 1992a), suggesting that either the renal tubular cells are less sensitive to the putative carcinogen(s) in cigarette smoke, or the exposure levels to these carcinogens is substantially lower in the kidney parenchyma.

Obesity

Obesity is another well-established risk factor for RCC. A body mass index (BMI) of 30 kg/m^2 (weight/height^2) has been consistently associated with a three- to sixfold increased risk of RCC in postmenopausal women and may account for up to 20% of kidney cancers in women (McLaughlin et al. 1984; Yu et al. 1986; Mellemgaard et al. 1995; Shapiro et al. 1999). Obesity does not appear to be as strong a risk factor for men, although studies have reported a two- to threefold increased risk for obese men compared with men of normal weight (Yu et al. 1986; Kreiger et al. 1993; Mellemgaard et al. 1995; Shapiro et al. 1999; Chow et al. 2000). Little is known about whether the rate of weight gain during adulthood or differences in body fat distribution are important factors in the development of RCC.

The mechanism by which obesity may increase RCC risk is not clear, but may relate to the increased exposure to oestrogens derived from an increase in adipose tissue (Longcope et al. 1986). Synthetic and natural oestrogens have been shown to increase DNA damage in the kidney and increase the risk of RCC in animals (Li et al. 1983; Hodgson et al. 1998). However, the evidence that hormone-associated factors (such as use of oral contraceptives or hormone replacement therapy, age at menarche and age at menopause) are associated with RCC in women is conflicting (McCredie and Stewart 1992a; Kreiger et al. 1993; Chow et al. 1995; Lindblad et al. 1995). Obesity may also increase the risk of RCC via other mechanisms associated with the insulin resistance syndrome, such as insulin-like growth factor-I (IGF-I) (Wolk et al. 1996b). However, little is known about the relationship between endogenous hormones and growth factors and the development of RCC.

Kidney disease

People with advanced kidney disease who undergo dialysis have a three to sixfold higher risk of RCC compared with healthy individuals (Inamoto et al. 1991; Buccianti et al. 1996; Maisonneuve et al. 1999). Other urinary tract disorders, such as kidney stones, cysts, urinary tract infections, tuberous sclerosis and other kidney injuries, have also been associated with an increased risk of RCC (McLaughlin et al. 1984; Maclure and Willett 1990; Washecka and Hanna 1991; McCredie and Stewart 1992a; Kreiger et al. 1993; Marple et al. 1994). From these data, it has been hypothesised that physical injury to the kidney or underlying renal disease places the organ at increased susceptibility to accumulated mutations during the carcinogenic process, although the precise mechanisms remain unclear.

Possible risk factors

Diet

Little is known about the role of diet in the development of RCC. An international correlation study found kidney cancer incidence and mortality rates to be associated with per-capita consumption of meat, fat and animal protein (Armstrong and Doll 1975). In addition, several case–control studies have found red meat to be associated with an increased risk of RCC (McLaughlin et al. 1984; Maclure and Willett 1990; Chow et al. 1994; De Stefani et al. 1998). In particular, well-done red meat has been implicated as a risk factor for RCC (Wolk et al. 1996b), possibly as a result of the generation of heterocyclic amines which can form DNA adducts in the kidney (Thorgeirsson et al. 1995). However, another study has not found such a relationship (Augustsson et al. 1999). Several case–control studies have found a high protein intake to be associated with an increased risk of RCC (Chow et al. 1994; De Stefani et al. 1998), although other studies have not confirmed this (Wolk et al. 1996b).

A diet rich in fruit and vegetables has been more consistently associated with a lower risk of RCC (Fraser et al. 1990; Maclure and Willett 1990; Negri et al. 1991; McLaughlin et al. 1992b; Wolk et al. 1996b; De Stefani et al. 1998). In particular, the antioxidant carotenoids, α-carotene, β-carotene, β-crytoxanthin and lutein, have been associated with a significant 30–40% reduced risk in a large US-based case–control study (Yuan et al. 1998a), although other studies have failed to find an association with intake of cruciferous vegetables (McLaughlin et al. 1984; Maclure and Willett 1990; Chow et al. 1994). RCC has not been associated with coffee, alcohol or any other beverage in case–control studies (Wolk et al. 1996a; Yuan et al. 1998a). More data are needed from large prospective studies to investigate whether dietary factors affect the development of RCC later in life.

Hypertension and antihypertensive medication

It has been suggested that the risk of RCC is increased by about two- to threefold if the patient has hypertension and/or uses hypertensive medication, such as diuretics. However, it is not clear from many of the epidemiological studies whether it is the underlying medical condition, the medications taken or the presence of kidney disease itself that accounts for this association.

In studies that have examined both diuretic use and hypertension, associations with these drugs independent of hypertension have been found, particularly among women (Yu et al. 1986; McLaughlin et al. 1988; Grove et al. 1991; Finkle et al. 1993; Kreiger et al. 1993; Hiatt et al. 1994). Conversely, an association with hypertension independent of diuretic use has also been reported (McCredie and Stewart 1992a; McLaughlin et al. 1995a; Chow et al. 1995; Shapiro et al. 1999). However, a recent cohort study in the USA found strong evidence of a dose–response relationship between blood pressure and RCC risk later in life, which lends further credence to the hypothesis that the condition rather than the treatment is associated with RCC

(Chow et al. 2000). The mechanism through which hypertension may increase RCC risk is unclear, although it may induce renal injury or be associated with metabolic changes within the renal tubules that increases susceptibility to carcinogens or exposure to promoting agents such as IGF-I (Cooper et al. 2001).

Analgesics

Phenacetin is an established cause of transitional cell tumours of the urinary tract (IARC 1987) and has been found to be a strong risk factor for cancer of the renal pelvis (McCredie et al. 1982, 1983a, 1983b; McLaughlin et al. 1983; Jensen et al. 1989). The role of phenacetin in the aetiology of RCC is less clear; a number of studies reported moderately elevated risks with regular or long-term use, but the low numbers of regular phenacetin users results in limited power to detect statistically significant associations (McLaughlin et al. 1984, 1985, 1992b; McCredie et al. 1988; Kreiger et al. 1993). In any case, the withdrawal of phenacetin-containing analgesics during the 1970s and 1980s in many Western countries means that phenacetin is unlikely to contribute to the development of many renal cell cancers today.

Few studies have investigated the association between other analgesics and RCC risk, despite the finding that high doses of aspirin and most other non-steroidal anti-inflammatory agents over the long term are associated with chronic renal dysfunction in both animals and humans (Perneger et al. 1994; D'Agati 1996). Although one case–control study in the USA found regular use of analgesics (of a dose higher than 325 mg/day) to be associated with a 2.5-fold increased risk for RCC in men and women (Gago-Dominguez et al. 1999), other large studies have found no such association (Lindblad et al. 1993; Mellemgaard et al. 1994; McCredie et al. 1995).

Occupational exposures

There has been no consistent association with type of employment and RCC, although, in some studies, occupational exposure to several known carcinogens, including asbestos, cadmium, polycyclic aromatic hydrocarbons, petrol and organic solvents, has been associated with an increased RCC risk (Mandel et al. 1995; Dosemeci et al. 1999; Pesch et al. 2000). However, other large studies have not confirmed these associations (Partanen et al. 1991; McLaughlin and Blot 1997; Sali and Boffetta 2000). If exposure to these chemicals is associated with an increased risk of RCC, it probably plays only a small role in the aetiology of this disease in the general population.

Potential for prevention

The incidence and mortality rates of kidney cancer have been rising steadily in most countries in recent years, a reflection of an increased detection of asymptomatic tumours and an increasing prevalence of obesity, smoking and hypertension, and possibly dietary changes. Given the relatively high attributable risks associated with lifestyle factors such as smoking and obesity, there is considerable potential for the prevention of RCC in many populations. Trends in incidence and, to a greater degree, mortality are therefore likely to improve substantially with implementation of public health policies that aim to stop smoking and reduce obesity in the general population.

Further research is urgently needed to understand the aetiology of RCC and to identify the mechanism(s) through which obesity and other factors influence cancer progression. The new generation of multicentre prospective studies provides a unique opportunity to explore the genetic, metabolic and nutritional determinants of this disease, which, if left at current trends, is set to become one of the major cancers of Western societies.

Acknowledgements

I am very grateful to Dr Timothy Key and Paul Appleby for helpful comments on the manuscript.

References

Armstrong B, Doll R (1975) Environmental factors and cancer incidence and mortality in different countries, with special reference to dietary practices. *International Journal of Cancer* **15**: 617–631.

Augustsson K, Skog K, Jagerstad M, Dickman PW, Steineck G (1999) Dietary heterocyclic amines and cancer of the colon, rectum, bladder, and kidney: a population-based study. *The Lancet* **353**: 703–707.

Buccianti G, Ravasi B, Cresseri D, Maisonneuve P, Boyle P, Locatelli F (1996) Cancer in patients on renal replacement therapy in Lombardy, Italy. *The Lancet* **347**: 59–60.

Chow WH, Gridley G, McLaughlin JK et al. (1994) Protein intake and risk of renal cell cancer. *Journal of the National Cancer Institute* **86**: 1131–1139.

Chow WH, McLaughlin JK, Mandel JS, Blot WJ, Niwa S, Fraumeni JF Jr (1995) Reproductive factors and the risk of renal cell cancer among women. *International Journal of Cancer* **60**: 321–324.

Chow WH, Devesa SS, Warren JL, Fraumeni JFJ (1999) Rising incidence of renal cell cancer in the United States. *Journal of the American Medical Association* **281**: 1628–1631.

Chow WH, Gridley G, Fraumeni JFJ, Jarvholm B (2000) Obesity, hypertension, and the risk of kidney cancer in men. *New England Journal of Medicine* **343**: 1305–1311.

Cooper ME, Bonnet F, Oldfield M, Jandeleit-Dahm K (2001) Mechanisms of diabetic vasculopathy: an overview. *American Journal of Hypertension* **14**: 475–486.

D'Agati V (1996) Does aspirin cause acute or chronic renal failure in experimental animals and in humans? *American Journal of Kidney Disease* **28**: S24–S29.

Damhuis RA, Kirkels W J (1998) Improvement in survival of patients with cancer of the kidney in Europe. EUROCARE Working Group. *European Journal of Cancer* **34**: 2232–2235.

De Stefani E, Fierro L, Mendilaharsu M et al. (1998) Meat intake, 'mate' drinking and renal cell cancer in Uruguay: a case-control study. *British Journal of Cancer* **78**: 1239–1243.

Dosemeci M, Cocco P, Chow WH (1999) Gender differences in risk of renal cell carcinoma and occupational exposures to chlorinated aliphatic hydrocarbons. *American Journal of Industrial Medicine* **36**: 54–59.

Ferlay J, Bray P, Pisani P, Parkin DM (2001) GLOBOCAN 2000: Cancer incidence, Mortality and Prevalence Worldwide, version 1.0. IARC CancerBase No. 5. Lyon, IARC Press. http:www-dep.iarc.fr/globocan.htm – accessed August 2001.

Finkle WD, McLaughlin JK, Rasgon SA, Yeoh HH, Low JE (1993) Increased risk of renal cell cancer among women using diuretics in the United States. *Cancer Causes and Control* **4**: 555–558.

Fraser GE, Phillips RL, Beeson WL (1990) Hypertension, antihypertensive medication and risk of renal carcinoma in California Seventh-Day Adventists. *International Journal of Epidemiology* **19**: 832–838.

Gago-Dominguez M, Yuan JM, Castelao JE, Ross RK, Yu MC (1999) Regular use of analgesics is a risk factor for renal cell carcinoma. *British Journal of Cancer* **81**: 542–548.

Gnarra JR (1998) von Hippel-Lindau gene mutations in human and rodent renal tumors – association with clear cell phenotype. *Journal of the National Cancer Institute* **90**: 1685–1687.

Grove JS, Nomura A, Severson RK, Stemmermann GN (1991) The association of blood pressure with cancer incidence in a prospective study. *American Journal of Epidemiology* **134**: 942–947.

Hiatt RA, Tolan K, Quesenberry CPJ (1994) Renal cell carcinoma and thiazide use: a historical, case-control study (California, USA). *Cancer Causes and Control* **5**: 319–325.

Hodgson AV, Ayala-Torres S, Thompson EB, Liehr JG (1998) Estrogen-induced microsatellite DNA alterations are associated with Syrian hamster kidney tumorigenesis. *Carcinogenesis* **19**: 2169–2172.

IARC (1986) *IARC Monographs on Evaluation for the Carcinogenic Risk of Chemicals to Humans: Tobacco smoking*, vol. 38. Lyon, France: International Agency for Research on Cancer.

IARC (1987) *Overall Evaluations of Carcinogenicity: An updating of IARC Monographs,* Vols 1–42, Suppl. 7. Lyon, France: International Agency for Research on Cancer.

Inamoto H, Ozaki R, Matsuzaki T, Wakui M, Saruta T, Osawa A (1991) Incidence and mortality patterns of malignancy and factors affecting the risk of malignancy in dialysis patients. *Nephron* **59**: 611–617.

Jensen OM, Knudsen JB, Tomasson H, Sorensen BL (1989) The Copenhagen case-control study of renal pelvis and ureter cancer: role of analgesics. *International Journal of Cancer* **44**: 965–968.

Kreiger N, Marrett LD, Dodds L, Hilditch S, Darlington GA (1993) Risk factors for renal cell carcinoma: results of a population-based case-control study. *Cancer Causes and Control* **4**: 101–110.

Lamiell JM, Salazar FG, Hsia YE (1989) von Hippel–Lindau disease affecting 43 members of a single kindred. *Medicine* **68**: 1–29.

Latif F, Tory K, Gnarra J, Yao M et al. (1993) Identification of the von Hippel-Lindau disease tumor suppressor gene. *Science* **260**: 1317–1320.

Li JJ, Li SA, Klicka JK, Parsons JA, Lam LK (1983) Relative carcinogenic activity of various synthetic and natural estrogens in the Syrian hamster kidney. *Cancer Research* **43**: 5200–5204.

Lindblad P, McLaughlin JK, Mellemgaard A, Adami H O (1993) Risk of kidney cancer among patients using analgesics and diuretics: a population-based cohort study. *International Journal of Cancer* **55**: 5–9.

Lindblad P, Mellemgaard A, Schlehofer B et al. (1995) International renal-cell cancer study. V. Reproductive factors, gynecologic operations and exogenous hormones. *International Journal of Cancer* **61**: 192–198.

Longcope C, Baker R, Johnston CCJ (1986) Androgen and estrogen metabolism: relationship to obesity. *Metabolism* **35**: 235–237.

Maclure M, Willett W (1990) A case-control study of diet and risk of renal adenocarcinoma, *Epidemiology* **1**: 430–440.

McCredie M, Stewart JH (1992a) Risk factors for kidney cancer in New South Wales, Australia. II. Urologic disease, hypertension, obesity, and hormonal factors. *Cancer Causes Control* **3**: 323–331.

McCredie M, Stewart JH (1992b) Risk factors for kidney cancer in New South Wales – I. Cigarette smoking, *European Journal of Cancer* **28A**: 2050–2054.

McCredie M, Ford JM, Taylor JS, Stewart JH (1982) Analgesics and cancer of the renal pelvis in New South Wales. *Cancer* **49**: 2617–2625.

McCredie M, Stewart JH, Ford JM (1983a) Analgesics and tobacco as risk factors for cancer of the ureter and renal pelvis. *Journal of Urology* **130**: 28–30.

McCredie M, Stewart JH, Ford JM, MacLennan R A (1983b) Phenacetin-containing analgesics and cancer of the bladder or renal pelvis in women. *British Journal of Urology* **55**: 220–224.

McCredie M, Ford JM, Stewart JH (1988) Risk factors for cancer of the renal parenchyma. *International Journal of Cancer* **42**: 13–16.

McCredie M, Pommer W, McLaughlin JK et al. (1995) International renal-cell cancer study. II. Analgesics. *International Journal of Cancer* **60**: 345–349.

McCredie M, Williams S, Coates M (1999) Cancer mortality in migrants from the British Isles and continental Europe to New South Wales, Australia 1975–1995. *International Journal of Cancer* **83**: 179–185.

McLaughlin JK, Blot W J (1997) A critical review of epidemiology studies of trichloroethylene and perchloroethylene and risk of renal-cell cancer. *International Archives of Occupational and Environmental Health* **70**: 222–231.

McLaughlin JK, Blot WJ, Mandel JS, Schuman LM, Mehl ES, Fraumeni JFJ (1983) Etiology of cancer of the renal pelvis. *Journal of the National Cancer Institute* **71**: 287–291.

McLaughlin JK, Mandel JS, Blot WJ, Schuman LM, Mehl ES, Fraumeni JFJ (1984) A population-based case-control study of renal cell carcinoma. *Journal of the National Cancer Institute* **72**: 275–284.

McLaughlin JK, Blot WJ, Mehl ES, Fraumeni JFJ (1985) Relation of analgesic use to renal cancer: population-based findings. *National Cancer Institute Monographs* **69**: 217–222.

McLaughlin JK, Blot WJ, Fraumeni JFJ (1988) Diuretics and renal cell cancer, *Journal of the National Cancer Institute* **80**: 378.

McLaughlin JK, Hrubec Z, Heineman EF, Blot WJ, Fraumeni JFJ (1990) Renal cancer and cigarette smoking in a 26-year follow-up of U.S. veterans. *Public Health Reports* **105**: 535–537.

McLaughlin JK, Silverman DT, Hsing AW et al. (1992a) Cigarette smoking and cancers of the renal pelvis and ureter. *Cancer Research* **52**: 254–257.

McLaughlin JK, Gao YT, Gao RN et al. (1992b) Risk factors for renal-cell cancer in Shanghai, China. *International Journal of Cancer* **52**: 562–565.

McLaughlin JK, Chow WH, Mandel JS et al. (1995a) International renal-cell cancer study. VIII. Role of diuretics, other anti-hypertensive medications and hypertension. *International Journal of Cancer* **63**: 216–221.

McLaughlin JK, Lindblad P, Mellemgaard A et al. (1995b) International renal-cell cancer study. I. Tobacco use, *International Journal of Cancer* **60**: 194–198.

McLaughlin JK, Blot WJ, Devesa SS (1996) Renal cancer. In: Schoffenfeld D, Fraumeni JF Jr (eds), *Cancer Epidemiology and Prevention,* 2nd edn. New York: Oxford University Press, pp. 1142–1155.

Maisonneuve P, Agodoa L, Gellert R et al. (1999) Cancer in patients on dialysis for end-stage renal disease: an international collaborative study. *The Lancet* **354**: 93–99.

Mandel JS, McLaughlin JK, Schlehofer B et al. (1995) International renal-cell cancer study. IV. Occupation. *International Journal of Cancer* **61**: 601–605.

Marple JT, MacDougall M, Chonko A M (1994) Renal cancer complicating acquired cystic kidney disease. *Journal of the American Society of Nephrology* **4**: 1951–1956.

Mellemgaard A, Niwa S, Mehl ES, Engholm G, McLaughlin JK, Olsen JH (1994) Risk factors for renal cell carcinoma in Denmark: role of medication and medical history. *International Journal of Epidemiology* **23**: 923–930.

Mellemgaard A, Lindblad P, Schlehofer B et al. (1995) International renal-cell cancer study. III. Role of weight, height, physical activity, and use of amphetamines. *International Journal of Cancer* **60**: 350–354.

Motzer RJ, Bander NH, Nanus D M (1996) Renal-cell carcinoma. *New England Journal of Medicine* **335**: 865–875.

Negri E, La Vecchia C, Franceschi S, D'Avanzo B, Parazzini F (1991) Vegetable and fruit consumption and cancer risk. *International Journal of Cancer* **48**: 350–354.

Neumann HP, Lips CJ, Hsia YE, Zbar B (1995) Von Hippel–Lindau syndrome. *Brain Pathology* **5**: 181–193.

Office for National Statistics (2001) Kidney. In: *Cancer Trends in England and Wales* 1950-1999. London: HMSO, pp. 60–65.

Partanen T, Heikkila P, Hernberg S, Kauppinen T, Moneta G, Ojajarvi A (1991) Renal cell cancer and occupational exposure to chemical agents. *Scandinavian Journal of Work and Environmental Health* **14**: 231–239.

Perneger TV, Whelton PK, Klag MJ (1994) Risk of kidney failure associated with the use of acetaminophen, aspirin, and nonsteroidal antiinflammatory drugs. *New England Journal of Medicine* **331**: 1675–1679.

Pesch B, Haerting J, Ranft U, Klimpel A, Oelschlagel B, Schill W (2000) Occupational risk factors for renal cell carcinoma: agent-specific results from a case–control study in Germany. MURC Study Group. Multicenter urothelial and renal cancer study. *International Journal of Epidemiology* **29**: 1014–1024.

Ries LAG, Eisner MP, Kosary CC et al. (2001) SEER Cancer Statistics Review 1973-1998. National Cancer Institute. Bethesda, MD. http://seer.cancer.gov/Publications/CSR1973-1998/ accessed August 2001.

Ross RK, Paganini-Hill A, Landolph J, Gerkins V, Henderson B E (1989) Analgesics, cigarette smoking, and other risk factors for cancer of the renal pelvis and ureter. *Cancer Research* **49**: 1045–1048.

Sali D, Boffetta P (2000) Kidney cancer and occupational exposure to asbestos: a meta-analysis of occupational cohort studies. *Cancer Causes Control* **11**: 37–47.

Schlehofer B, Pommer W, Mellemgaard A et al. (1996) International renal-cell-cancer study. VI. the role of medical and family history. *International Journal of Cancer* **66**: 723–726.

Schmidt L, Duh FM, Chen F et al. (1997) Germline and somatic mutations in the tyrosine kinase domain of the MET proto-oncogene in papillary renal carcinomas. *Nature Genetics* **16**: 68–73.

Shapiro JA, Williams MA, Weiss NS, Stergachis A, LaCroix AZ, Barlow WE (1999) Hypertension, antihypertensive medication use, and risk of renal cell carcinoma. *American Journal of Epidemiology* **149**: 521–530.

Smith SJ, Bosniak MA, Megibow AJ, Hulnick DH, Horii SC, Raghavendra BN (1989) Renal cell carcinoma: earlier discovery and increased detection. *Radiology* **173**: 699–703.

Thorgeirsson SS, Davis CD, Schut HA, Adamson RH, Snyderwine EG (1995) Possible relationship between tissue distribution of DNA adducts and genotoxicity of food-derived heterocyclic amines. *Princess Takamatsu Symposium* **23**: 85–92.

Washecka R, Hanna M (1991) Malignant renal tumors in tuberous sclerosis. *Urology* **37**: 340–343.

Wolk A, Gridley G, Niwa S et al. (1996a) International renal cell cancer study. VII. Role of diet. *International Journal of Cancer* **65**: 67–73.

Wolk A, Lindblad P, Adami HO (1996b) Nutrition and renal cell cancer. *Cancer Causes and Control* **7**: 5–18.

World Health Organization (2001) WHO Cancer Mortality Databank. http://www-dep.iarc.fr/dataava/globocan/who.htm – accessed August 2001.

Yu MC, Mack TM, Hanisch R, Cicioni C, Henderson BE (1986) Cigarette smoking, obesity, diuretic use, and coffee consumption as risk factors for renal cell carcinoma. *Journal of the National Cancer Institute* **77**: 351–356.

Yuan JM, Gago-Dominguez M, Castelao JE, Hankin JH, Ross RK, Yu MC (1998a) Cruciferous vegetables in relation to renal cell carcinoma. *International Journal of Cancer* **77**: 211–216.

Yuan JM, Castelao JE, Gago-Dominguez M, Yu MC, Ross RK (1998b) Tobacco use in relation to renal cell carcinoma. *Cancer Epidemiology Biomarkers, Prevention* **7**: 429–433.

Chapter 2

Identification of the individual at risk: the molecular and clinical genetics of renal cell carcinoma

Eamonn R Maher

Although only 2% of renal cell carcinoma (RCC) cases are familial, the elucidation of a genetic basis for inherited RCC has provided important insights into the mechanisms of renal tumorigenesis. In many cases specific genetic causes are associated with specific histopathological subtypes of RCC (Table 2.1). In addition to the disorders discussed here, RCC may also be a feature of hereditary non-polyposis colon cancer syndrome (Lynch and de la Chapelle 1999).

Genetic susceptibility to clear-cell renal cell carcinoma

von Hippel–Lindau disease

Von Hippel–Lindau (VHL) disease, a dominantly inherited multisystem familial cancer syndrome with an incidence of about 1 per 30 000, is the most frequent genetic cause of RCC susceptibility (Maher 1996).

Clinical features and diagnosis

The clinical presentation and course of VHL disease is very variable. The most common features are retinal haemangioblastomas (about 60% of cases), central nervous system (CNS) haemangioblastomas (about 60% of cases and usually in the cerebellum, although also in the spinal cord and brain stem and rarely supratentorially) and clear-cell RCC (Maher et al. 1990). Phaeochromocytoma occurs in about 10% of cases but there are marked interfamilial variations; in some kindreds this is the most common (or rarely the only) manifestation of VHL disease. Less common tumours include pancreatic endocrine neoplasms (often malignant but usually non-functional) and endolymphatic sac tumours (should be suspected if a VHL disease patient complains of deafness or tinnitus). Although renal, pancreatic and epididymal cysts are a common feature of VHL disease and may provide clues to the diagnosis, these are usually asymptomatic.

Clinical presentation of VHL may be in childhood or old age, but is most common between the ages of 15 and 40 years. Penetrance is almost complete by the age of 60 years, although RCC usually presents later than retinal and cerebellar haemangioblastomas. Thus, RCC is the presenting feature in about 10% of cases. The widespread introduction

Table 2.1 Inherited disorders in which RCC is a major feature

Disorder	Histopathology of RCC	Major associated tumours	Gene	Location
von Hippel–Lindau disease	Clear cell	Haemangioblastoma, phaeochromocytoma, pancreatic endocrine tumours	VHL	3p25
Chromosome 3 translocations	Clear cell		–	3p14–3q21
Familial clear-cell RCC	Clear cell		?	?
Hereditary papillary RCC	Type 1 papillary		MET	7q
Hereditary uterine leiomyomas and papillary RCC	Type 2 papillary	Leimyomas, leiomyosarcoma	FH	1q42–q44
Familial papillary thyroid cancer and papillary renal neoplasia	Papillary	Thyroid	?	1q21
Birt–Hogg–Dube syndrome	Oncocytoma (but variable)	Cutaneous fibrofolliculomas	BHD	17p11.2
Tuberous sclerosis	Variable	CNS hamartomas, renal angiomyolipomas	TSC1, TSC2	9q34, 16p13
Hyperpara-thyroidism–jaw tumour syndrome	Hamartoma Papillary		HRPT2	1q21–q31

of presymptomatic DNA testing and annual screening for asymptomatic tumours in gene carriers has significantly reduced the age at diagnosis. Interfamilial variations in the phenotypic expression of VHL disease reflect the differing tumour risks of specific VHL gene mutations (see Kaelin and Maher 1998). Most mutations produce a type 1 phenotype, which is characterised by the development of RCC, retinal and CNS haemangioblastomas, but not phaeochromocytoma. VHL type 2 subtypes are usually caused by missense mutations and are associated with phaeochromocytoma. Thus, VHL type 2A (which is rare in the UK) is characterised by phaeochromocytomas, retinal and CNS haemangioblastomas, but a low risk of RCC. Type 2B is characterised by phaeochromocytomas, RCC and CNS haemangioblastomas. Type 2C VHL disease is uncommon and manifests as familial phaeochromocytoma without other features of VHL disease. In the future, screening of asymptomatic VHL disease patients may be tailored according to the results of mutation analysis. However, intrafamilial phenotypic variability can result from stochastic events, genetic modifier effects and mosaicism (Webster et al. 1998; Sgambati et al. 2000).

Clinical criteria for the diagnosis of VHL disease require (1) a typical VHL tumour (e.g. haemangioblastoma, RCC or phaeochromocytoma) if there is a positive family history or (2) the presence of two tumours if there is no family history (e.g. two haemangioblastomas or a haemangioblastoma and a visceral tumour) (Maher et al. 1990). These criteria are reliable in most circumstances but recognition of isolated cases is delayed because of the need for two tumours to occur. Increasingly a suspected or clinical diagnosis of VHL disease is confirmed by molecular genetic analysis. Current VHL mutation analysis using a complete range of techniques can provide a detection rate approaching 100% in non-mosaic patients with classic VHL disease (Stolle et al. 1998). The uptake of predictive DNA testing by at-risk relatives is high because surveillance can be discontinued in those who are not gene carriers. Predictive testing is usually offered from the age of 5 years. In addition to establishing carrier status, VHL mutation characterisation may also provide clues to the likely phenotype (see above). Clinical and molecular investigations for VHL disease should be considered in all patients with familial, multicentric or early onset RCC.

Management and surveillance

The effective management of VHL disease requires a coordinated multidisciplinary approach. After the diagnosis of VHL disease in an index case, all at-risk relatives should be contacted and offered entry into a surveillance protocol (Table 2.2). Lifelong surveillance should be instigated for all gene carriers (irrespective of whether they are clinically affected).

Table 2.2 Example of a surveillance programme for von Hippel–Lindau disease in *asymptomatic* affected patients and at-risk relatives

Affected patient
1   Annual physical examination and urine testing
2   Annual direct and indirect ophthalmoscopy
3   MRI brain scan every 3 years to age 50 and every 5 years thereafter
4   Annual renal ultrasonography or MRI (CT may be required if multiple cysts renal or pancreatic cysts are present)
5   Annual 24-hour urine collection for catecholamines from age 11

At-risk relative
1   Annual physical examination and urine testing
2   Annual direct and indirect ophthalmoscopy from age 5 to 60 (fluorescein angioscopy or angiography may be used from age 10 to increase sensitivity)
3   MR brain scan every 3 years to from age 15 to 40 years and then every 5 years until age 60 years
4   Annual renal ultrasonography or MRI from age 15 to 65 years
5   Annual 24-hour urine collection for catecholamines from age 11

CT, computed tomography; MRI, magnetic resonance imaging.

The major renal manifestations of VHL disease are renal cystic disease and multiple, bilateral, clear-cell RCC. Although mean age at diagnosis of symptomatic RCC is about 40 years, the widespread adoption of surveillance programmes including annual renal imaging (Table 2.2) has resulted in many renal lesions being detected at an early stage. The surgical management of RCC in VHL disease is shifting from the treatment of large symptomatic RCC, to the challenge of managing small asymptomatic tumours. Most small renal tumours enlarge slowly (mean < 2 cm/year) and, after establishing the growth rate, an individual lesion can usually be scanned (by magnetic resonance imaging [MRI] or ultrasonography) every 6 months (Choyke et al. 1992). The risk of distant metastasis from a solid lesion < 3 cm appears to be remote and a non-interventional approach is usually followed until a tumour reaches a diameter of 3 cm when a limited partial nephrectomy is performed and other smaller encapsulated lesions are removed (Walther et al. 1999). Such a nephron-sparing approach suggests that, although the risk of local recurrence (from new primary tumours) is high, the risk of distant metastasis is low (Steinbach et al. 1995). In contrast, 25% of VHL disease patients with an RCC > 3 cm (treated by nephron-sparing surgery or nephrectomy) developed metastatic disease (Walther et al. 1999). A nephron-sparing approach to the management of RCC in VHL disease (and other forms of familial RCC) may, however, only delay the requirement for bilateral nephrectomy and renal replacement therapy in patients with bilateral multicentric disease. To date, experience with renal transplantation in VHL disease patients is encouraging and it appears that immunosuppression does not have adverse effects on the underlying course of VHL disease (Goldfarb et al. 1997).

Molecular genetics of VHL disease

The VHL gene functions as a tumour-suppressor gene such that inactivation of both alleles is required to initiate tumour development. In VHL disease patients, tumours retain the mutated VHL allele but the wild-type allele is inactivated by loss, mutation or methylation. Furthermore, about 60% of sporadic clear-cell RCCs demonstrate somatic inactivation of both VHL alleles (by loss, mutation or promoter methylation). Re-introduction of a wild-type VHL gene into sporadic clear-cell RCC cell lines with a defective VHL gene suppresses tumorigenicity (*pVHL*) (see Kaelin and Maher 1998; Clifford and Maher 2001). The precise mechanisms by which *pVHL* suppresses tumorigenesis is still under investigation. The VHL gene product is likely to have multiple functions and, in addition to regulating expression of a wide range of hypoxia-inducible mRNAs (see later), *pVHL* has been implicated in cell cycle control (Pause et al. 1998), fibronectin binding and extracellular matrix assembly (Ohh et al. 1998), and post-transcriptional regulation of target gene expression through mRNA stability effects (Gnarra et al. 1996; Knebelmann et al. 1998). VHL-related tumours are notably hypervascular and express high levels of vascular endothelial growth factor (VEGF) and other hypoxia-inducible mRNAs. Critical clues to the mechanism for this observation were provided by the recognition of structural similarities between a multimeric protein complex (the VCBCR complex), including *pVHL* and four other proteins (elongin C, elonginB, Cul2, Rbx1), and the SCF (Skp-1–Cdc53/Cul1-F box protein) class of E3 ubiquitin ligases (Lonergan et al. 1998). This observation suggested that the VCBCR complex may have a role in targeting oncogenic proteins for ubiquitin-dependent proteolysis (Pause et al. 1997; Lonergan et al. 1998). Subsequently pVHL was demonstrated to target the regulatory α subunits of hypoxia-inducible factors, HIF-1 and HIF-2, for oxygen-dependent proteolysis (Maxwell et al. 1999). HIF-1 is a heterodimeric transcription factor with a critical role in cellular responses to hypoxia. Under normoxic conditions, the HIF α subunits are degraded rapidly by the proteasome in a *pVHL*-dependent ubiquitylation process (Cockman et al. 2000). Constitutively high levels of HIF α subunits are observed in *VHL*-defective RCC lines, causing upregulation of an extensive range of hypoxia-inducible mRNAs, including those involved in energy metabolism, angiogenesis and apoptosis (e.g. GLUT-1 and VEGF). Thus the association of *pVHL* with HIF-1 regulation provides an explanation for the vascularity of VHL-related tumours.

Chromosome 3 translocations and clear-cell RCC

An important, albeit rare, cause of susceptibility to clear-cell RCC is a pericentromeric chromosome 3 translocation; this should be excluded in all cases of familial, multicentric or early onset clear-cell RCC. The first report of an association between clear-cell RCC and a chromosome 3 translocation [(t(3;8)(p14;q24)] in a large Italian American kindred suggested an RCC susceptibility gene at 3p14 (Cohen et al. 1979). Translocation carriers developed bilateral or multiple tumours, with a penetrance of 67%. Subsequently an increased risk of thyroid cancer was also reported in the family. Further reports of chromosome 3 translocations associated with RCC susceptibility described a variety of chromosome 3 breakpoints, e.g. t(3;6)(p13;q25) (Kovacs et al. 1989), t(2;3)(q35;q210) (Bodmer et al. 1998) and t(3;12)(q35;q21) (Kovacs and Hoene 1988), so it was uncertain whether there was a specific RCC suppressor gene at 3p14. In a classic tumour-suppressor gene model, it would be predicted that RCC from t(3;8)(p14;q24) gene carriers would retain the derivative (translocated) chromosome 3 and lose the normal chromosome 3 (so that both copies of a 3p14 tumour-suppressor gene would be inactivated). However, analysis of tumours from patients with the t(3;8) [and also t(3;6) and t(2;3)] RCC-associated translocations demonstrate loss of the derivative chromosome 3 and retention of the normal chromosome 3. In addition, the VHL allele on the retained normal chromosome 3 is mutated (the VHL allele on the derivative chromosome is lost), so that the tumours are defective for the VHL tumour-suppressor gene (Schmidt et al. 1995; Bodmer et al. 1998).

Thus, it is thought that the pericentromeric chromosome 3 translocation associated with RCC may cause tumour susceptibility, not because a particular gene is disrupted but because the derivative chromosome 3 is liable to be lost by random non-disjunction.

Translocation carriers in kindreds with chromosome 3 translocations and RCC should be offered regular renal surveillance as for VHL disease (see above). There are relatively few data available for the risk of RCC in patients ascertained after the finding of a chromosome 3 translocation, although one study suggested a substantially increased risk of RCC in translocation carriers (van Kessel et al. 1999).

Familial, non-VHL, clear-cell RCC

The definition of subtypes of familial RCC based on histopathology and the availability of molecular genetic testing for germline *VHL* and *MET* gene mutations have led to the recognition of families with dominantly inherited susceptibility to clear-cell RCC who do not have VHL disease or a chromosome 3 translocation (Teh et al. 1997; Woodward et al. 2000). The molecular basis of familial, non-VHL, clear-cell RCC (FCRC) has not been defined, but FCRC is not allelic with VHL disease and does not map to chromosome 3p (Teh et al. 1997; Woodward et al. 2000). Age at onset of RCC is variable in FCRC and, although, on average, RCC may develop later than in VHL disease, screening by renal imaging should be offered to at-risk relatives from the age of 20 years in kindreds with early onset cases (Woodward et al. 2000). To date there is no evidence of a significantly increased risk for non-renal cancers in FCRC kindreds.

Genetic susceptibility to non-clear cell RCC

Hereditary papillary RCC type 1 (HPRC1)

Papillary RCC is the most common form of non-clear-cell RCC. Recently, it was suggested that papillary RCC can be subdivided into two groups: type 1 tumours, which are usually multiple and low grade, and type 2, which are single, of higher grade and have a poorer prognosis (Delahunt and Eble 1997). Familial papillary RCC is a rare, dominantly inherited disorder (minimum prevalence 1 per 10^7) characterised by the development of multiple, bilateral papillary RCCs. Hereditary papillary RCC (HPRC) is caused by germline mutations in the *MET* proto-oncogene (Zbar et al. 1995; Schmidt et al. 1997). The germline *MET* gene mutations detected are missense and appear to be activating mutations within the tyrosine kinase domain (Schmidt et al. 1997). Non-penetrance is common and there is a high frequency of subclinical disease in gene carriers who undergo renal imaging. Individuals with, or at risk for, HPRC1 should be offered annual renal imaging from the age of 30 years. Patients with germline *MET* gene mutations and *HPRC1* have type 1 tumours, so the histopathological analysis can be used to guide the priority for molecular genetic investigation (Lubensky et al. 1999).

Hereditary uterine leiomyomas and papillary RCC

This recently described disorder is characterised by dominantly inherited susceptibility to uterine leiomyomas, type 2 papillary renal cancers and cutaneous nodules (leiomyomas) (Launonen et al. 2001). The hereditary leiomyomatosis and renal cancer gene maps to chromosome 1q and results from heterozygous mutations in fumarate hydratase (FH).

Birt–Hogg–Dube syndrome

Birt–Hogg–Dube syndrome (BHD) is a dominantly inherited disorder characterised by the development, usually in the third or fourth decade, of multiple cutaneous papules distributed over the face, neck and upper trunk. Histological examination of the skin lesions reveals fibrofolliculomas, trichodiscomas and acrochordomas. Spontaneous pneumothorax and lipoma are also features and there may be an increased risk of colorectal polyps. Recently, an association between BHD and renal tumours was described (Toro et al. 1999). Although BHD was initially recognised in some kindreds with familial oncocytoma (Weirich et al. 1998), other histological subtypes have been described in BHD kindreds. In view of the elevated risk of RCC in some BHD kindreds, it is suggested that affected individuals should be offered annual renal ultrasound scans from the age of 25 years.

A BHD gene maps to chromosome 17p11.2 (Schmidt et al. 2001) and interestingly, a naturally occurring familial kidney cancer in dogs, renal cystadenocarcinoma and nodular dermatofibrosis, may be an animal model for BHD (Jonasdottir et al. 2000). The BHD gene encodes a protein, folliculin, of unknown function (Nickerson et al. 2002).

Tuberous sclerosis

This dominantly inherited multiple hamartoma syndrome has been associated with an increased risk of RCC, although angiomyolipomas are the most common renal tumour in tuberous sclerosis (Sampson et al. 1995; Al-Saleem et al. 1998). Tuberous sclerosis is caused by germline mutations in the *TSC1* and *TSC2* tumour-suppressor genes. In rats, germline mutations in *TSC2* cause the Eker rat model of familial non-clear-cell RCC (Kobayashi et al. 1995). Nevertheless, it appears that RCC is infrequent in tuberous sclerosis, although there are several reports of multifocal and bilateral disease in young patients (Sampson et al. 1995; Al-Saleem et al. 1998).

Familial papillary thyroid cancer and papillary renal neoplasia

Malchoff et al. (2000) described a kindred with familial papillary thyroid cancer susceptibility mapping to chromosome 1q21. Two family members developed papillary renal tumours, suggesting a common link between these tumour types.

Hyperparathyroidism–jaw tumour syndrome

A familial hyperparathyroidism syndrome associated with jaw cysts (hyper-parathroidism–jaw tumour syndrome [HPT-JT]) was mapped to chromosome 1q21-q31 by Szabo et al. (1995). Subsequently, Teh et al. (1996) confirmed this mapping and reported an association with renal cysts and hamartomas. Recently, Haven et al.

(2000) described a further family linked to the HPT-JT region in which a variety of tumours, including renal cortical adenoma and papillary RCC, were associated with parathyroid tumours and renal cysts. The HPRT2 gene was identified recently and encodes the parafibromin gene product (Carpten et al. 2002).

Conclusion

The recognition and appropriate management of kindreds with familial renal cancer are important because of the opportunities for reducing morbidity and mortality. Key pieces of information in reaching a precise diagnosis include (1) the histopathology of the renal tumours, (2) the presence or absence of associated extrarenal tumours, and (3) the nature of any associated cutaneous lesions. Cytogenetic (for a chromosome 3 translocation) and molecular genetic testing (e.g. for *VHL* and *MET* mutations as appropriate) can further inform the diagnosis. When a diagnosis is reached, at risk relatives should be identified and offered appropriate screening.

References

Al-Saleem T, Wessner LL, Scheitauer BW et al. (1998) Malignant tumours of the kidney, brain and soft malignant tissues in children and young adults with the tuberous sclerosis complex. *Cancer* **83**: 2208–2216.

Bodmer D, Eleveld MJ, Ligtenberg MJL et al. (1998) An alternative route for multistep tumorigenesis in a novel case of hereditary renal cell cancer and a t(2;3)(q35;q21) chromosome translocation. *American Journal of Human Genetics* **62**: 1475–1483.

Carpten JD, Robbins CM, Villablanca A et al. (2002) HRPT2, encoding parafibromin, is mutated in hyperparathyroidism-jaw tumor syndrome. *Nature Genetics* **32**(4): 676–680.

Choyke PL, Glenn GM, Walther MCM et al. (1992) The Natural-History of Renal Lesions in von Hippel–Lindau Disease – a Serial CT Study in 28 Patients. *American Journal of Roentgenology* **159**: 1229–1234.

Clifford SC, Maher ER (2001) Von Hippel–Lindau disease: clinical and molecular perspectives. *Advances in Cancer Research* **82**: 85–105.

Cockman ME, Masson N, Mole DR et al. (2000) Hypoxia inducible factor-alpha binding and ubiquitylation by the von Hippel–Lindau tumor suppressor protein. *Journal of Biological Chemistry* **275**: 25733–25741.

Cohen AJ, Li FP, Berg S et al. (1979) Hereditary renal cell carcinoma associated with a chromosomal translocation. *New England Journal of Medicine* **301**: 592–595.

Delahunt B, Eble JN (1997) Papillary renal cell carcinoma: a clinicopathologic and immunohistochemical study of 105 tumors. *Modern Pathology* **10**: 537–544.

Gnarra JR., Zhou S, Merrill MJ et al. (1996) Post-transcriptional regulation of vascular endothelial growth factor mRNA by the product of the VHL tumor suppressor gene. *Proceedings of the National Academy of Science of the USA* **93**: 10589–10594.

Goldfarb DA, Neumann HP, Penn I, Novick AC (1997) Results of renal transplantation in patients with renal cell carcinoma and von Hippel–Lindau disease. *Transplantation* **64**: 1726–1729.

Haven CJ, Wong FK, van Dam EW et al. (2000) A genotypic and histopathological study of a large Dutch kindred with hyperparathyroidism-jaw tumor syndrome. *Journal of Clinical Endocrinology and Metabolism* **85**: 1449–1454.

Jonasdottir TJ, Mellersh CS, Moe L et al. (2000) Genetic mapping of a naturally occurring hereditary renal cancer syndrome in dogs. *Proceedings of the National Academy of Science of the USA* 97: 4132–7.

Kaelin WG, Maher ER (1998) The VHL tumour suppressor gene paradigm. *Trends in Genetics* **14**: 423–425.

Knebelmann B, Ananth S, Cohen HT, Sukhatme VP (1998) Transforming growth factor alpha is a target for the von Hippel–Lindau tumor suppressor. *Cancer Research* **58**: 226–231.

Kobayashi T, Hirayama Y, Kobayashi E, Kubo Y, Hino O (1995) A germline insertion in the tuberous sclerosis (Tsc2) gene gives rise to the Eker rat model of dominantly inherited cancer. *Nature Genetics* **9**: 70–74.

Kovacs G, Hoene E (1988) Loss of der(3) in renal carcinoma cells of a patient with constitutional t(3;12). *Human Genetics* **78**: 148–150.

Kovacs G, Brusa P, De Riese W (1989) Tissue-specific expression of a constitutional 3;6 translocation: development of multiple bilateral renal-cell carcinomas. *International Journal of Cancer* **43**: 422–427.

Launonen V, Vierimaa O, Kiuri M et al. (2001) Inherited susceptibility to uterine leiomyomas and renal cell cancer. *Proceedings of the National Academy of Science of the USA* **98**: 3387–3392.

Lonergan KM, Iliopoulos O, Ohh M et al. (1998) Regulation of hypoxia-inducible mRNAs by the von Hippel-Lindau tumor suppressor protein requires binding to complexes containing elongins B/C and Cul2. *Molecular and Cellular Biology* **18**: 732–741.

Lubensky IA, Schmidt L, Zhuang, ZP et al. (1999) Hereditary and sporadic papillary renal carcinomas with c-*MET* mutations share a distinct morphologic phenotype. *American Journal of Pathology* **155**: 517–526.

Lynch HT, de la Chapelle A (1999) Genetic susceptibility to non-polyposis colorectal cancer. *Journal of Medical Genetics* **36**: 801–818.

Maher ER (1996) Inherited renal cell carcinoma. *British Journal of Urology* **78**: 542–545.

Maher ER, Yates JRW, Harries R et al. (1990) Clinical features and natural history of von Hippel–Lindau disease. *Quarterly Journal of Medicine* 77: 1151–1163.

Malchoff CD, Sarfarazi M, Tendler B et al. (2000) Papillary thyroid carcinoma associated with papillary renal neoplasia: genetic linkage analysis of a distinct heritable tumor syndrome. *Journal of Clinical Endocrinology and Metabolism* **85**: 1758–1764.

Maxwell PH, Wiesener MS, Chang GW et al. (1999) The tumour suppressor protein VHL targets hypoxia-inducible factors for oxygen-dependent proteolysis. *Nature* **399**: 271–275.

Nickerson ML, Warren MB, Toro JR et al. (2002) Mutations in a novel gene lead to kidney tumors, lung wall defects, and benign tumors of the hair follicle in patients with the Birt-Hogg-Dube syndrome. *Cancer Cell* **2**(2): 157–164.

Ohh M, Yauch RL, Lonergan KM et al. (1998) The von Hippel–Lindau tumor suppressor protein is required for proper assembly of an extracellular fibronectin matrix. *Molecular Cell* 1: 959–968.

Pause A, Lee S, Worrell RA et al. (1997) The von Hippel–Lindau tumor-suppressor gene product forms a stable complex with human CUL-2, a member of the Cdc53 family of proteins. *Proceedings of the National Academy of Science of the USA* **94**: 2156–2161.

Pause A, Lee S, Lonergan KM, Klausner RD (1998) The von Hippel–Lindau tumor suppressor gene is required for cell cycle exit upon serum withdrawal. *Proceedings of the National Academy of Science of the USA* **95**: 993–998.

Sampson JR, Patel A, Mee AD (1995) Multifocal renal cell carcinoma in sibs from a chromosome 9 linked (TSC1) tuberous sclerosis family. *Journal of Medical Genetics* **32**: 848–850.

Schmidt L, Li F, Brown RS et al. (1995) Mechanism of tumorigenesis of renal carcinomas associated with the constitutional chromosome 3;8 translocation. *Cancer Journal of the Scientific American* **1**: 191–196.

Schmidt L, Duh FM, Chen F et al. (1997) Germline and somatic mutations in the tyrosine kinase domain of the MET proto-oncogene in papillary renal carcinomas. *Nature Genetics* **16**: 68–73.

Schmidt LS, Warren MB, Nickerson ML et al. (2001) Birt–Hogg–Dube syndrome, a genodermatosis associated with spontaneous pneumothorax and kidney neoplasia, maps to chromosome 17p11.2. *American Journal of Human Genetics* **69**: 876–882.

Sgambati MT, Stolle C, Choyke PL et al. (2000) Mosaicism in von Hippel–Lindau disease: lessons from kindreds with germline mutations identified in offspring with mosaic parents. *American Journal of Human Genetics* **66**: 84–91.

Steinbach F, Novick AC, Zincke H et al. (1995). Treatment of renal-cell carcinoma in von Hippel–Lindau disease – a multicenter study. *Journal of Urology* **153**: 1812–1816.

Stolle C, Glenn G, Zbar B et al. (1998) Improved detection of germline mutations in the von Hippel–Lindau disease tumor suppressor gene. *Human Mutations* **12**: 417–423.

Szabo J, Heath B, Hill VM, Jackson CE et al. (1995) Hereditary hyperparathyroidism–jaw tumor syndrome: the endocrine tumor gene HRPT2 maps to chromosome 1q21–q31. *American Journal of Human Genetics* **56**: 944–950.

Teh BT, Farnebo F, Kristoffersson U et al. (1996) Autosomal dominant primary hyper-parathyroidism and jaw tumor syndrome associated with renal hamartomas and cystic kidney disease: linkage to 1q21–q32 and loss of the wild type allele in renal hamartomas. *Journal of Clinical Endocrinology and Metabolism* **81**: 4204–4211.

Teh BT, Giraud S, Sari NF et al. (1997) Familial non-VHL non-papillary clear-cell renal cancer. *The Lancet* **349**: 848–849.

Tomlinson IP, Alam NA, Rowan AJ et al. (2002) Germline mutations in FH predispose to dominantly inherited uterine fibroids, skin leiomyomata and papillary renal cell cancer. *Nature Genetics* **30**(4): 406–410.

Toro J, Duray P, Glenn G et al. (1999) Birt–Hogg–Dube syndrome: a novel marker of renal neoplasia. *Archives in Dermatology* **135**: 1195–1202.

van Kessel AG, Wijnhoven H, Bodmer D et al. (1999) Renal cell cancer: chromosome 3 translocations as risk factors. *Journal of the National Cancer Institute* **91**: 1159–1160.

Walther MM, Choyke PL, Glenn G et al. (1999) Renal cancer in families with hereditary renal cancer: Prospective analysis of a tumor size threshold for renal parenchymal sparing surgery. *Journal of Urology* **16**: 1475–1479.

Webster AR, Richards FM, MacRonald FE, Moore AT, Maher ER (1998) An analysis of phenotypic variation in the familial cancer syndrome von Hippel–Lindau disease: Evidence for modifier effects. *American Journal of Human Genetics* **63**: 1025–1035.

Weirich G, Glenn G, Junker K et al. (1998) Familial renal oncocytoma: clinicopathologic study of 5 families. *Journal of Urology* **160**: 335–340.

Woodward ER, Clifford SC, Astuti D, Affara NA, Maher ER (2000) Familial clear cell renal cell carcinoma (FCRC): clinical features and mutation analysis of the VHL, MET, and CUL2 candidate genes. *Journal of Medical Genetics* **37**: 348–353.

Zbar B, Glenn G, Lubensky I et al. (1995) Hereditary papillary renal cell carcinoma: clinical studies in 10 families. *Journal of Urology* **153**: 907–912.

Chapter 3

Current thinking on the natural history of and prognostic factors in renal cell cancer

R Tim D Oliver

Although it has long been known (Everson and Cole 1966) that renal cancer has one of the higher frequencies (Table 3.1), there has been considerable controversy regarding how often spontaneous regression actually occurs. Bloom (1973) estimated that it was 0.3% from a literature review, whereas Werf-Messing (1971), from a personal series of 35 metastatic renal cancer patients observed without treatment, reported that 30% showed non-progression at 6 months. This polarity of view and the increasing recognition of the impact of patient selection on outcome of treatment (de Kernion et al. 1978) prompted the author to set out to investigate prospectively its frequency in the setting of the good performance status patients referred to tertiary centres who undertake clinical trials. An increasingly recognised characteristic of trials in renal cell cancer was that initial reports were often double that achieved when the treatment became generally available. As a result of this, there was an increased need to exclude the possibility that the responses reported for biological treatment simply reflected episodes of spontaneous regression in the highly selected subgroup referred to these specialist centres.

In order to investigate this further, patients with early but asymptomatic metastases underwent a period of surveillance to investigate what was the frequency of spontaneous regression and whether there was any relationship between spontaneous regression and response to cytokine therapy. It is the aim of this chapter to review the results of this study (Oliver et al. 1988, 1989; Oliver 1989) and their relevance to modern treatment of cancer.

Overview of spontaneous tumour rejection in renal cancer and possible common mechanisms

In the 30 years since Everson and Cole (1966) first published that spontaneous regression of cancer was a real entity, there have been more than 70 cases reported (Fairlamb 1981) and four major attempts (Bloom 1973; Gleave et al. 1998; Oliver et al. 1988; Possinger et al. 1988) to estimate the frequency (Table 3.2). The first by Bloom (1973), although detecting a frequency of only 0.3% in the retrospective literature review, did report 2 of 172 (1.2%) in Bloom's own personal series. An update of this retrospective overview was reported by Possinger et al. (1988). In that report of 1247 patients, only 0.24% showed spontaneous regression. It was 2.5 times higher

Table 3.1 Spontaneous regression of cancer (Challis and Stam 1990)

	No. of cases
Leukaemia/Lymphoma	121
Melanoma	69
Renal cell cancer	68
Neuroblastoma	41
Gastrointestinal cancer	34
Retinoblastoma	33
Lung	25
Breast	22
Testis	16
Other	75
Total	504

in the 50% of patients with sufficiently good performance status to enable nephrectomy to be performed. Both prospective studies (Oliver et al. 1988; Gleave et al. 1998) report a much higher incidence of spontaneous regression (7.1% and 6.1%). The latter was the most interesting because these cases were the control arm of a randomised double-masked trial with placebo injections given to the controls who all had a reasonable performance status. Today, our own prospective phase II surveillance study has recruited 292 patients with 13 unexplained regressions, and an additional 9 patients with prolonged stable disease. Although the regression rate in the initial personally treated series was 7%, with increased numbers and a wider range of doctors seeing the patients, the response rate has declined to 4.5% in the more recently treated series (Table 3.3). These last series also coincided with the advent of interleukin-2 (IL2) and a trend to less delay if there was any suspicion of progression. The limited analysis performed seems to confirm the previously reported association with performance status, site of metastasis (i.e. lung vs other) (Table 3.4) and the presence or absence of hypercalcaemia (Oliver et al. 1988).

Table 3.2 'Unexplained' regression in renal cell cancer

	No. of cases	'Unexplained' regression (%)
Metastases all (Possinger et al. 1988)	1247	0.24
Post-nephrectomy (Possinger et al. 1988)	663	0.6
Personal series (Bloom 1973)	172	1.2
Oliver et al. (1988)	72	7.1
Placebo injections, randomised trial (Gleave et al. 1998)	99	6.1

Table 3.3 'Spontaneous' regressions prolonged stable disease in
St Bartholomew's and Royal London Renal Cell Cancer Surveillance Studies

Study		No. of cases	CR + PR + SD (%)
Retrospective	Before 1978	55	0 + 2 + NA
Prospective	1978–85	73	4 + 3 + 6
Prospective	1986–93	91	0 + 4 + 6
Prospective	1994–98	73	0 + 4 + 3
Total		292	1 + 3 + 3

CR, complete response; NA, not applicable; PR, partial response; SD, stable disease.

Table 3.4 'Spontaneous' regression with response to subsequent therapy in
patients with metastatic renal cancer

	No. of cases	CR (%)	PR (%)	OR (%)
Total surveillance series	292	1	3	3
Lung metastases only	71	8	5	13
Others	221	0	2	2
Entered into cytokine studies after progression on surveillance	132	3	8	16
Lung metastases only	23	14	30	50
Others	109	0	2	2

As far as mechanisms are concerned, it has been assumed to have some sort of immunological basis, although a non-immunological anti-angiogenic effect has by no means been excluded. Two of the thirteen patients in this department's studies have features that would fit with an immunological mechanism (Oliver 1989). The first was a patient who had a regression, which lasted nearly 4 years. It began after her husband, who was a violent alcoholic, dried out and stopped beating her. Her metastases regrew when his alcoholism returned and then regressed again when she left him, but then recurred after 3 years and she ultimately died at 4 years. The concept of chronic stress-related immunosuppression accelerating tumour growth has been well documented in experimental animal models (Temoshok et al. 1985) and supported by observations from breast cancer (Spiegel et al. 1989). The second case was an example of the rarely reported (Ritchie et al. 1988) spontaneous regression of liver metastases. The history given by the patient suggested that the regression may have been caused by viral oncolysis in vivo. Eight years before presentation the patient had had a nephrectomy and had been well until about 4 weeks before he was first seen. He had just returned from Indonesia where he had developed an acute episode of swinging fever, nausea and vomiting, which had continued when he returned home. As he got so progressively ill, he was investigated and found to have an enlarged liver with elevated enzymes. A computed tomography (CT) scan showed that nearly a third of the liver was replaced by metastases and biopsy confirmed clear-cell carcinoma. Within one week of biopsy he began to feel better, paralleled by a reduction in hepatomegaly and an improvement in liver enzymes, which slowly returned to normal after about 8 weeks. By 3 months his CT scan was nearly normal and remained so for 10 months when he relapsed and died within 12 weeks, with an enlarging liver, but no other metastases, totally unresponsive to cytokines or chemotherapy. Although viral antibody titres to known hepatitis-causing viruses were negative, it was concluded that he had probably been infected with an obscure south-east Asian hepatitis virus which had induced viral oncolysis, as has been demonstrated using the Newcastle disease virus (Lindenmann and Klein 1967; Schirrmacher et al. 1989).

Although these studies of surveillance have proved to be safe, the frequency of response in this highly selected group of tertiary referrals was less than that seen from cytokine treatment. The response rate after progression on surveillance differed little from that reported by other authors. However, as it is the same group of good-risk patients with small volume lung metastases developing late or being present at the time of nephrectomy who respond to cytokines and show spontaneous regression (see Table 3.4), there is some degree of anxiety that surveillance could prejudice response. Currently, our policy is to use a brief period of surveillance before entry into cytokine trials, to get an assessment of their disease progression rate and assess for psychological factors contributing to tumour progression, and it is continued only in patients who are obviously improving.

Comparison of response to therapy after exclusion of spontaneous regression with literature reports

The overall results from our sequential phase II studies undertaken with patients progressing after surveillance (Table 3.5) was somewhat less (unless stable disease lasting more than 3 months in our more advanced poor-risk population is regarded as a response category) than reported in the major overviews of published series (Table 3.6). All of our studies have been with subcutaneous IL2 and some authors have suggested that results have been better after high-dose intravenous schedules. Table 3.7 summarises recent large phase II series and demonstrates that there is no obvious benefit from intravenous compared with subcutaneous treatments. In addition more is not necessarily better in terms of total dose. The published response rate of renal cell cancer metastases to interferon-α is somewhat less than that to IL2. However, given the degree of selection for good-risk patients in the IL2 studies because of worry about cardiac risks, it is unlikely that the difference is of any significance because the survival of and incidence in long-term disease-free survivors is the same. The lack of any advantage for the higher-dose continuous intravenous infusion route of administration over the lower-dose subcutaneous regimens has obvious economic benefits, although it will be important to wait for the report on the long-term follow-up of the randomised low- versus high-dose intravenous versus subcutaneous IL2 study currently being run though the US National Cancer Institute (Table 3.7) before the issue is closed.

Table 3.5 Royal London phase II studies in metastatic RCC (Oliver et al. 1999)

	No. of cases	CR (%)	PR (%)	OR (%)	MR/SD (%)
BCG	19	10	5	15	15
Interferon-α	21	0	13	13	13
IL2	25	4	8	12	12
IL/IFNα	24	0	0	0	2
IL/IFNα/5FU	43	2	12	14	21
Total	132	3	8	11	16

CR, complete response; 5FU, 5-fluorouracil; IFN, interferon; IL, interleukin; PR, partial response; OR, overall response; MR/SD, minor response/stable disease > 3 months.

Table 3.6 Overview of cytokine phase II studies in metastatic renal cell cancer

Cytokine	No. of cases	CR (%)	PR (%)	OR (%)
IFNα alone	1100	2	14	16
IL2 alone (i.v.)	848	5	11	16
IL2 alone (s.c.)	146	3	21	24
IL2 + IFNα i.v.	121	7	18	25
IL2 + IFNα s.c.	513	6	15	21
IL2/IFNα/5FU	313	7	26	33

CR, complete response; 5FU, 5-fluorouracil; IFN, interferon; IL, interleukin; i.v., intravenous; PR, partial response; OR, overall response; s.c., subcutaneous.

Table 3.7 Schedule and response of metastatic renal cancer to IL2

Dose (mu) schedule	Route	Total dose	No. of cases	CR + PR (%)
18/9 x 5/week for 4 weeks	s.c.	279	116	4 + 10
3 twice daily x 5/week for 6 weeks	s.c.	180	92	2 + 19
19/9 x 5/week for 6 weeks	s.c.	315	53	5.5 + 5.5
5 three times daily x 5/week for 1–2 weeks	i.v.	61	55	0 + 4
50 three times daily x 5/week for 1–2 weeks	i.v.	605	56	7 + 9
36 x 5/week for 2 weeks	c.i.v.	342	225	3.5 + 8.5

CR, complete response; PR, partial response.

The lack of more than an extremely marginal difference between IL2 and IL2 plus interferon-α (IFNα) (see Table 3.6) could be more significant than the lack of difference between IL2 and IFNα because the selection criteria for the former studies were similar. This issue is of some importance given what looks at first glance like a substantial advantage for the latest combination to be reported, i.e. 5-flurouracil (5FU) with IL2 and IFNα. However, not all of the centres that have so far reported on this regimen have had such a high response to the three-drug IFNα/IL2/5FU regimen (Table 3.8). In the study of Joffe et al. (1996), if patients who had not been nephrectomised were excluded, the response rate was similar to that of Atzpodien who originated the somewhat complicated regimen (Lopez Hanninen et al. 1996). This was not true in our series (Table 3.8) because one of the best responses was in a patient with extensive bone metastases who remains progression free at 3 years. However, from a clinical point of view there was little doubt that there was more substantial clinical benefit in poor-risk patients than in previous series using monotherapy. This translated into the fact that 21% of patients demonstrated major durable (> 6 months) clinical benefit with improved performance status off treatment, even though they did not achieve consideration of adequate shrinkage as a definite measurable response.

Table 3.8 Interferon-a/interleukin-2/5-flurouracil in metastatic renal cell cancer

Reference	No. of cases	CR (%)	PR (%)	OR (%)
Atzpodien in Lopez Hanninen et al. (1996)	120	11	28	39
Sella (1995); Ellerhorst et al. (1997)	46	8	35	43
Hofmockel et al. (1996)	34	9	29	38
Vaughan et al. (1997)	21	-	38	38
Joffe et al. (1996)	55	-	16	16
Oliver et al. (1999)	37	3	11	14
Herpen et al. (2000)	51	0	12	12

CR, complete response; PR, partial response; OR, overall response

Furthermore, there was one other new dimension that emerged from this study which could help go a long way to understanding why some centres report a better response than others. There was a higher response rate the further the patient had to travel, and the lowest response rate was observed in our local patients (Oliver et al. 1999). There is increasing recognition of the role of poverty in leading to a poor outcome from cancer treatment, most notably in the outcome of breast cancer. In our own centre (Oliver 2000) where the same degree of difference in survival is demonstrated if our surgeons operate on people referred in from regions with a high cure rate as are visible in the cancer registry figures, it is clear that this difference is not the result of poorer provision of surgical care. There is increasing evidence from studies of the effect of poverty on resistance to infectious disease that vitamin A enhances CD4 T-cell immune responses (Semba et al. 1993), vitamin D enhances CD8 T-cell and macrophage function (Koga et al. 1999; Veldman et al. 2000), and zinc enhances general immune response (Umeta et al. 2000). There is evidence from several cancers for the importance of vitamin A deficiency in accelerating cancer deaths, although importantly, in respect of cancer prevention trials, there is no benefit from supplements in individuals with already adequate levels of dietary intake (Hunter et al. 1993). There is also evidence from studies of breast and prostate cancer for the importance of vitamin D (Hanchette and Schwartz 1992). In addition there are data showing that vitamin D suppresses production of metalloprotease which plays a major role in tumour invasion (Koli and Keski-Oja 2000). These observations suggest that more attention will need to be paid to the issue of poverty in assessing response to treatments in the future.

Survival and randomised cytokine trials

Despite the big difference in response, as yet there is less evidence from studies of survival than from studies of response to suggest a higher survival rate after combination therapy than after monotherapy. In our own studies, though, there is a non-significant difference in survival at 12 months between the 46 most recently treated patients receiving IFNα/IL2/5FU and the historic series of 58 receiving monotherapy before 1995 (28% vs 16%). However, the difference narrowed when survival of 22 concurrent patients, unfit for the three-drug regimen, who had their recurrence treated with interferon alone, was examined (20%). Clearly only a randomised trial examining monotherapy versus the three-drug regimen will resolve the issue of whether there is survival advantage. With two randomised trials, one comparing non-cytokine therapy versus monotherapy and one versus the three-drug combination, both showing significant relapse-free and overall survival advantage for cytokine therapy (Table 3.9), but with the only trial of monotherapy versus dual IFN plus IL2 showing progression-free albeit not overall survival advantage, the proposed MRC trial comparing monotherapy versus triple therapy is extremely timely.

Relevance of spontaneous regression to and effect of lead-time bias on prognostic factor analysis

Since the landmark study of de Kernion et al. (1978), it is well established that selection can have a powerful effect on outcome. This is equally relevant to the incidence of spontaneous regression (Oliver et al. 1988). It is these observations that make it difficult to exclude the fact that selection and lead-time bias play a part in the apparent benefit of cytokine therapy.

Table 3.9 Randomised cytokine trials in renal cancer cells

Trial	Reference	Response in control area	Response in therapy area
MPA vs IFNα	Steinbeck et al. (1990)	28%[a] (n = 30)	28%[a] (n = 30)
MPA vs IFNα	MRC (1998)	31%[a] (n = 168)	43%* (n = 167)
Placebo vs IFNγ	Gleave et al. (1998)	7%[c] (n = 90)	4%[b] (n = 91)
Tamoxifen vs IFNα/IL2	Henriksson et al.	3%[b] (n = 63)	8%[b] (n = 68)
Tamoxifen vs IFNα/IL2	Negrier et al. (1996)	7%[c] (n = 138)	19%[c] (n = 140)
Tamoxifen vs IFNα/IL2/5FU	Atzpodien et al. (2000)	0%[c] 14 months+[d] (n = 38)	33% > 42 months+[d] (n = 41)

[a]1-year survival.
[b]Complete response.
[c]Overall response.
[d]Median survival.
5FU, 5-fluorouracil; IFNa, interferon-a; IFNg, interferon-g; IL2, interleukin-2; MPA, medroxyprogesterone acetate.

It is well recognised that lead-time bias from early diagnosis is a major problem for interpreting the results of radical prostatectomy (Dennis and Resnick 2000). The few studies that have investigated the impact of early diagnosis from increased availability of ultrasonography, intravenous urography (IVU) and CT scans on prognosis of renal cancer have, as yet, not demonstrated any evidence for population-based change in survival. There are several anecdotal reports demonstrating that, if renal tumours are diagnosed incidentally at time of angiography or ultrasonography for a non-malignant disease investigation, the prognosis is apparently better in terms of a lower frequency of metastases (Thompson and Peek 1988; Mevorach et al. 1992). However, this does not make allowance for two factors. First, such cases are obviously diagnosed long before they would present clinically, i.e. there is a lead-time bias. Second, if one does a postmortem examination on people dying of other causes, many more renal cancers are found than are actually detected clinically and a proportion of these even have metastases (Table 3.10).

Access to ultrasonography for diagnosis of renal cell cancer is substantially less available in the UK compared with Germany, where it is available in GP's surgeries. As a result, a higher proportion of British patients have unresectable primary

Table 3.10 Postmortem detection of 'occult' renal cell cancer

Number of autopsies	16 294
Total renal cell cancers	350 (2%)
Unrecognised RCC pre mortem	235 (67%)
Unrecognised RCC M+	56 (23%)

tumours. Given these observations, it is easy to understand why the two British unselected series of cases treated with the IFNα/IL2/5FU regimen demonstrated substantially less obvious advantage of the three-drug regimen (see Table 3.8).

It may be concluded that, at present, evidence that treatment actually reduces population-based mortality is still in doubt. It could be clouded by lead-time bias and over-diagnosis of small tumours, with small amounts of metastases that could be accelerated by surgery, and then be more susceptible to response to treatment, thus ending up with a survival neutral effect.

New approaches to prognostic factor analysis using simple peripheral blood parameters

There is increasing evidence that several peripheral blood parameters, such as erythrocyte sedimentation rate (ESR), pre-treatment platelet count and granulocyte count, post-treatment lymphocytosis (Table 3.11) and pre-treatment haemoglobin (Table 3.12), may predict for overall patient response and survival, although to date no single series has been large enough to do a multivariate analysis to separate them out. However, clinically they make an extremely interesting group of factors because they provide an insight into an even larger area of biology of renal cancer.

For many years ESR was the only way to monitor disease activity in patients with tuberculosis and, as such, it probably gave a good indication of the degree of disarray of immune response to the bacterium. Little work has been done on this parameter in recent years; it is certainly worth re-examining in the face of these new data, and also in the light of the observation that the response of the acute phase reactant, C-reactive protein, after treatment can serve as a prognosticator for response (Deehan et al. 1994).

Both IL6 and vascular endothelial growth factor (VEGF) have been identified as tumour products that could be involved in causing increased levels of platelets. With increasing interest and new clinical trials on compounds that block tumour angiogenesis (Cao et al. 1998; Browder et al. 2000), study of the molecular basis of platelet over-production could provide important information in the near future.

There is increasing recognition that over-production of granulocyte colony-stimulating factor (G-CSF) and granulocyte–macrophage CSF (GM-CSF) is a common oncofetal change detected in tumour cell lines in vitro (particularly bladder), and is associated with a poor outcome (Ito et al. 1990; Ohigashi et al. 1992). A similar effect may explain why a high neutrophil count is a poor prognostic feature in renal cancer patients. Both G-CSF and GM-CSF are the product of mesenchymal cells. In renal cell cancer mesenchymal elements, i.e. spindle cell or sarcomatoid change, are associated with a poor prognosis. It will be important to investigate this correlation further because its simplicity makes it easier than measurement of serum levels of G-CSF and GM-CSF.

Table 3.11 Haematological indices and response to low-dose subcutaneous interleukin-2

ESR	No. of cases	Response (%)
< 20	11	55
20–50	39	28
> 50	42	10

Response to IL2	No. of cases	Degree of lymphocytosis (%)
CR + PR	21	163
SD	37	67
PD	34	28

Platelets	No. of cases	1-year survival (%)
< 338 x 10^9/l	16	48
> 338 x 10^9/l	17	11

Platelets	No. of cases	Mean survival (months)
< 4 x 10^5/ml	112	34
< 4 x 10^5/ml	147	18

CR, complete response; ESR, erythrocyte sedimentation rate; PR, partial response; SD, stable disease.

Table 3.12 Interaction between haemoglobin status and response to interferon

	Response at 6 months (CR + PR + SD) (%)		Median progression free		Hazard ratio
	MPA	Interferon	MPA	Interferon	MPA vs interferon
All cases	14	23	2.75	3.50	0.66
Low Hb	5	10	2.00	2.00	0.79
Mid Hb	15	19	2.75	3.00	0.70
High Hb	21	46	2.75	6.50	0.51

CR, complete response; Hb, haemoglobin; MPA, medroxyprogesterone acetate; PR, partial response; SD, stable disease.

In contrast to the poor prognostic association with a raised neutrophil count is the good prognostic effect of an elevated lymphocytosis induced by IL2 (see Table 3.11). It is surprising that, despite the large number of studies of IL2, few have commented on this parameter, which seems in the one study where it has been systematically examined to be a powerful predictor that needs to be assessed prospectively in association with induction of autoimmune thyroiditis, another immunological parameter that predicts a good outcome (Franzke et al. 1999). It could be worth collecting cases of spontaneous regression worldwide to see how many of them also manifest any of these immune characteristics after rejection of their metastases.

That low haemoglobin was associated with a poorer outcome has been well established for several cancers, and in cervix cancer transfusing up to a normal level has been shown to improve survival in one study (Grogan et al. 1999). In general it is not thought to add much more to the general effect of poor performance status from widespread, poorly differentiated, malignant tumour. However, in renal cancer, admittedly so far only from one study involving 370 patients, there has emerged an even more interesting observation in relation to elevated haemoglobin level. This study (see Table 3.12) was a randomised trial comparing medroxyprogesterone acetate and IFNα. There was a higher response rate and better survival for those with haemoglobin in the upper third; moreover only those with haemoglobin levels in the upper third showed significant response and survival benefit from treatment with IFN. Erythropoietin is a normal differentiation product of renal cells and its production by a proportion of renal cancers is well established. This observation could be a demonstration that more differentiated, less clonally evolved tumours are the ones that respond to immunotherapy, as has been demonstrated by the high response of early bladder cancer to BCG (Bacille Calmette–Guérin).

A suggestion that it may result from more than being a marker of differentiation comes from an in vitro study which demonstrated that transfection of an erythropoietin gene into a non-secreting tumour enhanced susceptibility to immune T lymphocytes (Miyajima et al. 1996). The observed association of the clear-cell phenotype with erythropoietin production is therefore very interesting because the results from the small pilot study of allo-peripheral blood stem cell grafts (Childs et al. 2000) suggested that most of the responding patients had clear cell phenotype (9 of 12 clear cell vs 1 of 7 mixed tumours responded). The final possible factor that might be involved is anoxia because erythropoietin is produced in response to anoxia (Gleadle and Ratcliffe 1997), and such tumours could then be considered to lack adequate vascularisation and be very susceptible to anti-angiogenic drugs.

As all these parameters can be assessed on a single blood sample, they offer a very simple approach to prognostication. Understanding their mechanism of action could potentially offer insight into a wide perspective of cell biology. However, they fall into two groups: first those that increase the chance of response to immune therapy, i.e. lymphocytosis, induction of autoimmune response on therapy or high haemoglobin pre-treatment. The second group are mainly paraneoplastic inappropriate switches such as anaemia induced by G-CSF, IL6 and VEGF, which presumably indicate poorly differentiated cancers. These observations need to be investigated in large databases using multivariate analysis to establish whether they are independently significant or linked prognostic factors. They also need to be compared retrospectively in series of patients who have undergone spontaneous regression.

Prognostic factor analysis and need for adjuvant and neoadjuvant studies before surgery

There are small amounts of data (Lopez Hanninen et al. 1996), admittedly from serial phase II studies, that suggest that patients with a good prognosis have a greater gain from the three drugs IFNα/IL2/5FU when compared with the two-drug combination (IFNα/IL2). If this is real, it could well be that there is even more benefit from use of these drugs in the early stages of diseases. This is one of the observations that is justifying the current European Organisation for Research and Treatment of Cancer (EORTC) adjuvant study in patients with a poor risk, defined on the basis of the pathological criteria of vascular invasion and tumour size (Ravi and Oliver 1999). This is at present recruiting rather slowly but, given the increasing importance of the question it is asking, there is a clear need to focus more on this issue as a priority.

The reports of two studies with a benefit from nephrectomy in the face of metastases before starting interferon (Flanigan et al. 2000; Mickisch et al. 2000) are encouraging. However, there have been several reports that demonstrate that a sizeable minority, varying from 9% to 40% of metastatic disease patients, are not suitable for such studies because they are either inoperable or after a nephrectomy they progressed so rapidly that they become unfit for treatment (Fleischmann and Kim 1991; Rackley et al. 1994; Bennett et al. 1995; Franklin et al. 1996; Walther et al. 1997). This observation raises the question of whether it might be better to give cytokines as a preoperative neoadjuvant treatment. One phase II study has reported encouraging results from this approach in terms of tumour down-staging and overall survival from surgery (Kim and Louie 1992). In a second study, it was possible to generate tumour-infiltrating lymphocytes for therapy (Figlin et al. 1997). A randomised trial comparing pre- versus postsurgery cytokines is needed to clarify the value of this approach. Given the long-standing debate about the value of radical versus limited surgery in cancer, this will be an important trial. It is long been accepted that in breast cancer, super-radical mastectomy does not improve the results over mastectomy (Lacour et al. 1983). That the same may apply to radical prostatectomy remains subjudice despite the negative Veterans' trial (Iversen et al. 1995), until we get the results of the Scandinavian trial.

There are several observations that contribute to understanding why radical surgery may accelerate metastatic growth, so that the gain from extended surgery is undermined by its acceleration of metastases and local recurrence. Minimising these factors by tumour down-staging could be the potential gain from the experimental arm of the proposed trial of pre- versus postsurgery cytokines.

The first potential reversible effect of surgery is the immunosuppressive effect of anaesthesia, which has been well established from studies of phytohaemagglutinin-induced lymphocytes before and after surgery (Riddle and Berenbaum 1967). The immunosuppression after anaesthesia is at least as strong as azothiaprine, the principal drug used to immunosuppress transplant recipients, and its degree is proportional to the duration of anaesthesia.

The second factor is the impact of the handling effect on the tumour at the time of surgery. Studies in patients undergoing radical prostatectomy using reverse transcription polymerase chain reaction (RT-PCR) have demonstrated showers of tumour cell activity in the blood after surgery (Eschwege et al. 1995). Given that renal call cancer is one of the most vascular of all tumours, and that there are now markers to detect renal cancer cells in the circulation (Taille et al. 2000), the same sort of data could be produced by renal vein sampling at the time of nephrectomy. Comparing the number of cells in the renal vein at the time of surgery in the proposed pre- versus postsurgery cytokine study could be an interesting surrogate endpoint to justify the study.

The third factor undermining the effect of radical surgery is tumour acceleration induced by cytokines in the process of tissue repair. This has been known about since the time of Peyton Rous (Rous and Beard 1935), but there was relatively little attention paid to this issue, despite confirmatory data published by Alexander et al. (1988) who demonstrated a potential way of preventing its deleterious effects using anti- epithelial growth factor (EGF) antibody.

The fourth factor is renal-specific growth factors, the existence of which is demonstrated by the occurrence of compensatory hypertrophy of the contralateral kidney after unilateral nephrectomy.

Despite this myriad of potentially confounding tumour-accelerating effects of surgery, there is still uncertainty about whether they really play a sufficiently important role in the actual clinical situation in the cancer patient to justify attention. However, the evidence that immune-related treatments work better on the early stages of clonal evolution does justify a pre- versus postsurgery cytokine trial that could enable a prospective investigation of these perioperative issues.

It may be concluded that, at present, evidence that treatment of renal cell cancer actually reduces population-based mortality survival is still in doubt. It could be clouded by lead-time bias, leading to over-diagnosis of small tumours with small amounts of metastases, which could be accelerated by surgery and then be more susceptible to response to treatment, ending up with a survival neutral effect. To resolve this, there is a need to investigate whether animal data that demonstrate that use of an antibody to block EGF receptor prevents tumour implantation at sites of tissue repair apply clinically. If the proposed pre- versus postsurgery cytokine trial is successful, it could be followed by a randomised trial to investigate the use of the anti-EGF approach. Resolving this long-standing issue could be of relevance to the use of surgery at several tumour sites. Another issue that might be of relevance to examine in such trials is the role of laparoscopic surgery (Walther et al. 1999, because potentially such surgery might reduce some of the tumour-accelerating factors discussed above.

Conclusion

As an increasing number of studies are now confirming, it is clear that spontaneous regression of metastatic renal cancer occurs in 4–6% of patients eligible for cytokine trials, in which response rates of 12–18% are reported. Furthermore, as with cytokine-induced responses, spontaneous regression is more frequent in good-risk patients with small volumes of metastatic disease. There is as yet little formal proof that the same immunological mechanisms are involved in both types of response. However, the strongest anecdotal evidence for T cells being involved comes from a single case report of spontaneous regression of established metastases after reversion of immunosuppression after treatment of HIV disease with anti-HIV therapy (Morris 2000), and less unequivocally from reports of regressions occurring after relief of major psychological stress and after an episode of postulated, acute, non-specific, viral hepatitis-induced viral oncolysis. With evidence from three sources (i.e. melanoma HLA-B7 gene therapy study, study of haemoglobin production by renal cancer, and use of BCG and cytokines in bladder cancer) highlighting the view that immunosurveillance and immune-related therapies function most effectively in clonal early cancer, there is a clear need to develop research trials that examine the role of such treatments in the perioperative setting.

A proposal for a pre- versus post-nephrectomy cytokine study in patients presenting with already established metastases has been outlined as one approach to investigate this issue. The evidence that level of lymphocyte response to cytokines and degree of autoimmunity induced by therapy are predictors of chance of response to cytokines is increasingly firm. Furthermore, there is increasing recognition of the importance of normal expression of HLA class 1 antigen expression in tumours responding to immunological treatments (Ransom et al. 1992; Nouri et al. 1998). These observations suggest that the current ongoing attempts to develop vaccines for renal cell cancer could benefit from study of immunological basis of autoimmunity and the antigenic determinants that are the targets for the response.

References

Alexander P, Murphy P, Skipper D (1988) Preferential growth of blood borne cancer cells at site of trauma – a growth promoting role of macrophages. *Advances in Experimental Medicine and Biology* **233**: 245–251.

Bennett R, Lerner S, Taub H, Dutcher J, Fleischmann J (1995) Cytoreductive surgery for stage IV renal cell carcinoma. *Journal of Urology* **154**: 32–34.

Bloom HJ (1973) Hormone-induced and spontaneous regression of metastatic renal cancer. *Cancer* **32**: 1066–1071.

Browder T, Butterfield C, Kraling B et al. (2000) Antiangiogenic scheduling of chemotherapy improves efficacy against experimental drug-resistant cancer. *Cancer Research* **60**: 1878–1886.

Cao Y, O'Reilly M, Marshall B, Flynn E, Ji R, Folkman J (1998) Expression of angiostatin cDNA in a murine fibrosarcoma suppresses primary tumour growth and produces long-term dormancy of metastases. *Journal of Clinical Investigation* **101**: 1055–1063.

Challis GB, Stam HJ (1990) Spontaneous regression of cancer: a review of cases 1900–1987. *Acta Oncologica* **29**: 545–550.

Childs R, Chernoff A, Contentin N (2000) Regression of metastatic renal cell carcinoma after nonmyeloablative allogenic peripheral blood stem cell transplantation. *New England Journal of Medicine* **343**: 750–758.

Deehan D, Heys S, Simpson W, Herriot R, Broom J, Eremin O (1994) Correlation of serum cytokine and acute phase reactant levels with alterations in weight and serum albumin in patients receiving immunotherapy with recombinant IL-2. *Clinical and Experimental Immunology* **95**: 366–372.

de Kernion JB, Ramming KP, Smith RB (1978) The natural history of metastatic renal cell carcinoma: a computer analysis. *Journal of Urology* **120**: 148–152.

Dennis L, Resnick M (2000) Analysis of recent trends in prostate cancer incidence and mortality. *Prostate* **42**: 247–252.

Ellerhorst J, Sella A, Amato R et al. (1997) Phase II trial of 5-fluorouracil, interferon-alpha and continuous infusion interleukin-2 for patients with metastatic renal cell carcinoma. *Cancer* **80**: 2128–2132.

Eschwege P, Dumas F, Blanchet P et al. (1995) Haematogenous dissemination of prostatic epithelial cells during radical prostatectomy. *The Lancet* **346**: 1528–1529.

Everson TC, Cole WH (1966) *Spontaneous Regression of Cancer*. Philadelphia: WB Saunders.

Fairlamb D (1981) Spontaneous regression of metastases of renal cancer: A report of two cases including the first recorded regression following irradiation of a dominant metastasis and review of the world literature. *Cancer* **47**: 2102–2106.

Figlin RA, Pierce WC, Kaboo R et al. (1997) Treatment of metastatic renal cell carcinoma with nephrectomy, interleukin-2 and cytokine-primed or CD8(+) selected tumor infiltrating lymphocytes from primary tumor. *Journal of Urology* **158**: 740–745.

Flanigan R, Blumenstein B, Salmon S, Crawford E (2000) Cytoreduction nephrectomy in metastatic renal cancer: The results of Southwest Oncology Group Trial 8949. *Proceedings of the American Society for Oncology* **19**(suppl): abstract 3.

Fleischmann J, Kim B (1991) Interleukin-2 immunotherapy followed by resection of residual renal cell carcinoma. *Journal of Urology* **145**: 938–941.

Franklin J, Figlin R, Rauch J, Gitlitz B, Belldegrun A (1996) Cytoreductive surgery in the management of metastatic renal cell carcinoma: the UCLA experience. *Seminars in Urology and Oncology* **14**: 230–236.

Franzke A, Peest D, Probst-Kepper M et al. (1999) Autoimmunity resulting from cytokine treatment predicts long-term survival in patients with metastatic renal cell cancer. *Journal of Clinical Oncology* **17**: 529–533.

Gleadle, J, Ratcliffe, P (1997) Induction of hypoxia-inducible factor-1, erythropoietin, vascular endothelial growth factor, and glucose transporter-1 by hypoxia: evidence against a regulatory role for Src kinase. *Blood* **89**: 503–509.

Gleave ME, Elhilali M, Fraydet Y et al. (1998) Interferon gamma-1b compared with placebo in metastatic renal cell carcinoma. *New England Journal of Medicine* **338**: 1265–1271.

Grogan M, Thomas GM, Melamed I et al. (1999) The importance of hemoglobin levels during radiotherapy for carcinoma of the cervix. *Cancer* **86**: 1528–1536.

Hanchette, C, Schwartz, G (1992) Geographic patterns of prostate cancer mortality: evidence for a protective effect of ultraviolet radiation. *Cancer* **70**: 2861–2869.

Herpen C von, Jansen R, Kruit W et al. (2000) Immunochemotherapy with interleukin-2, interferon-alpha and 5-fluorouracil for progressive metastatic renal cell carcinoma: a multicentre phase II study. Dutch Immunotherapy Working Party. *British Journal of Cancer* **82**: 772–776.

Hofmockel G, Langer W, Theiss M (1996) Immunochemotherapy for metastatic renal cell carcinoma using a regimen of interleukin-2, interferon-a and 5-fluorouracil. *Journal of Urology* **156**: 18–21.

Hunter DJ, Manson JE, Colditz GA et al. (1993) A prospective study of the intake of vitamins C,E and A and the risk of breast cancer. *New England Journal of Medicine* **329**: 234–240.

Ito N, Matsuda T, Kakchi Y, Takeuchi E, Takashi T, Yoshida O (1990) Bladder cancer producing granulocyte colony stimulating factor. *New England Journal of Medicine* **323**: 1709–1710.

Iversen P, Madsen PO, Corle DK (1995) Radical prostatectomy versus expectant treatment for early carcinoma of the prostate. Twenty-three year follow-up of a prospective randomized study. *Scandinavian Journal of Urology and Nephrology* **172**(suppl): 65–72.

Joffe J, Banks R, Forbes M et al. (1996) A phase II study of interferon-alpha, interleukin-2 and 5-fluorouracil in advanced renal carcinoma: clinical data and laboratory evidence of protease activation. *British Journal of Urology* **77**: 638–649.

Joynes F, Rouse P (1914) On the cause of localisation of secondary tumours at points of injury. *Journal of Experimental Medicine* **20**: 404–412.

Kim B, Louie AC (1992) Surgical resection following interleukin-2 therapy for metastatic renal cell carcinoma prolongs remission. *Archives of Surgery* **127**: 1343–1349.

Koga Y, Naraparaju V, Yamamoto N (1999) Antitumour effect of vitamin D-binding protein derived macrophage activating factor on Ehrlich ascites tumour-bearing mice. *Proceedings of the Society for Experimental Biology and Medicine* **220**: 20–26.

Koli K, Keski-Oja J (2000) 1 alpha, 25-dihydroxyvitamin d3 and its analogues down-regulate cell invasion-associated proteases in cultured malignant cells. *Cell Growth Differentiation* **11**: 221–229.

Lacour J, Le M, Caceres E, Koszarowski T, Veronesi U, Hill C (1983) Radical mastectomy versus radical mastectomy plus internal mammary dissection. Ten year results of an international cooperative trial in breast cancer. *Cancer* **51**: 1941–1943.

Lindenmann J, Klein PA (1967) Viral oncolysis: increased immunogenicity of host cell antigen associated with influenza virus. *Journal of Experimental Medicine* **126**: 93–108.

Lopez Hanninen E, Kirchner H, Atzpodien J (1996) Interleukin-2 based home therapy of metastatic renal cell carcinoma: risks and benefits in 215 consecutive single institution patients. *Journal of Urology* **155**: 19–25.

Mevorach R, Segal A, Tersegno M, Frank I (1992) Renal cell carcinoma: Incidental diagnosis and natural history: Review of 235 cases. *Urology* **39**: 519–522.

Mickisch G, Garin A, Madej M, Prijck L, Sylvester R. de (2000) Tumour nephrectomy plus interferon alpha is superior to interferon alpha alone in metastatic renal cell carcinoma. *Journal of Urology* **163**(suppl): 778 (abstract).

Miyajima J, Imai Y, Nakao M, Noda S, Itoh K (1996) Higher susceptibility of erythropoietin-producing renal cell carcinomas to lysis by lymphokine-activated killer cells. *Journal of Immunotherapy With Emphasis On Tumor Immunology* **19**: 399–404.

Morris D (2000) Dramatic response of renal cell carcinoma to epivir and viramune in a HIV positive patient. *Proceedings of the American Society of Clinical Oncology* **18**(suppl).

Nouri A, Oliver R, Nagund V (1998) Clonal development of bladder cancer and its relevance to the clinical potential of HLA antigen and p53 based gene therapy. *Cancer Surveys* **31**: 109–128.

Ohigashi T, Tachibana M, Tazaki H, Nakamura K (1992) Bladder cancer cells express functional receptors for granulocyte–colony stimulating factor. *Journal of Urology* **147**: 283–286.

Oliver RTD (1989) Psychological support for cancer patients. *The Lancet* **ii**: 1209.

Oliver RTD (2000) Poorer outcome from treatment of breast cancer in poorer areas of Glasgow. *British Medical Journal* **408**: 321.

Oliver RTD, Miller RM, Mehta A, Barnett MJ (1988) A phase 2 study of surveillance in patients with metastatic renal cell carcinoma and assessment of response of such patients to therapy on progression, *Molecular Biotherapy* **1**: 14–20.

Oliver RTD, Nethersall ABW, Bottomley JM (1989) Unexplained spontaneous regression and alpha-interferon as treatment for metastatic renal carcinoma. *British Journal of Urology* **63**: 128–131.

Oliver RTD, Steele J, Ansell W (1999) Should spontaneous regression be excluded before commencing biotherapy in renal cancer? *British Journal of Urology International* **83**(suppl 4): 137 (abstract).

Possinger K, Wagner H, Beck R, Staebler A (1988) Renal cell carcinoma. *Controversies in Oncology* **30**: 195–207.

Rackley R, Novixk A, Klein E, Bukowski R, McLain D, Goldfarb D (1994) The impact of adjuvant nephrectomy on multimodality treatment of metastatic renal cell carcinoma. *Journal of Urology* **152**(5 pt 1): 1399–1403.

Ransom J, Pelle B, Hanna M (1992) Expression of class II major histocompatability complex molecules correlates with human colon tumour vaccine efficacy. *Cancer Research* **52**: 3460–3466.

Ravi R, Oliver RTD (1999) Recent progress in cytokine therapy for renal cell cancer. The case for the EORTC adjuvant cytokine trial in patients with poor risk renal cell cancer after maximum debulking surgery. *British Journal of Urology* **83**: 219–227.

Riddle P, Berenbaum M (1967) Postoperative depression of the lymphocyte response to phytohaemagglutinin. *The Lancet* **i**: 746–748.

Ritchie A, Layfield L, de Kernion J (1988) Spontaneous regression of liver metastases from renal carcinoma. *Journal of Urology* **140**: 596–597.

Schirrmacher V, von Hoegen P, Schlag P, Liebrich W, Lehner B, Schumaker K (1989) Active specific immunotherapy with autologous tumor cell vaccines modified by Newcastle disease virus: experimental and clinical studies. In *Cancer Metastasis* (V. Schirrmacher, R. Schwartz-Albiez eds) pp.157–170. Springer Verlag, Berlin, Heidelberg, New York.

Semba, R, Muhilal, Ward, B et al. (1993) Abnormal T cell subset proportions in Vitamin A deficient children. *The Lancet* **341**: 5–8.

Spiegel, D, Bloom, J, Kraemer, H, Gottheil, E (1989) Effect of psychosocial treatment on survival in patients with metastatic breast cancer. *The Lancet* **ii**: 888–891.

Taille, AdL, Cho Y, Shabsigh, A et al. (2000) Potential diagnostic significance of blood based RT–PCR assays of MN/CA9 and PSMA. *Journal of Urology* **163**: (abstract 686).

Temoshok L, Peeke HVS, Mehard CW, Axelsson K, Sweet SM (1985) Stress–behaviour interactions in hamster tumor growth. *Neuroimmune Interactions* **496**: 501–509.

Thompson I, Peek, M (1988) Improvement in survival of patients with renal cell carcinoma – The role of the serendipitously detected tumour. *Journal of Urology* **140**: 487–490.

Umeta M, West C, Haidar J, Deurenberg P, Hautvaset J (2000) Zinc supplementation and stunted infants in Ethiopia: a randomised controlled trial. *The Lancet* **355**: 2021–2026.

Vaughan M, Johnson S, Moore J (1997) A phase II study of subcutaneous interleukin-2, alpha interferon and prolonged venous infusional 5 FU in metastatic renal cell cancer. *British Journal of Cancer* **76**(suppl I): 50.

Veldman C, Cantorna M, DeLuca H (2000) Expression of 1,25-dihydroxyvitamin D (3) receptor in the immune system. *Archives of Biochemistry and Biophysics* **374**: 334–338.

Walther M, Yang J, Pass H, Linehan W, Rosenberg S (1997) Cytoreductive surgery before high dose interleukin-2 based therapy in patients with metastatic renal cell carcinoma. *Journal of Urology* **158**: 1675–1678.

Walther M, Lyne J, Libutti S, Linehan W (1999) Laparoscopic cytoreductive nephrectomy as preparation for administration of systemic interleukin-2 in the treatment of metastatic renal cell carcinoma: a pilot study. *Urology* **53**: 496–501.

Werf-Messing VD (1971) Hormonal treatment of metastases of renal carcinoma. *British Journal of Cancer* **25**: 423–427.

PART 2

Histopathology and imaging

Defining the role of pathology services in the diagnosis and staging of renal cell carcinoma

Alexander J Howie

Pathologists contribute to the management of renal cell carcinoma (RCC) by answering three questions. First, is the diagnosis renal cell carcinoma, rather than something else? Second, what type of renal cell carcinoma is it? Third, what features are present that are of relevance to prognosis?

Is the diagnosis renal cell carcinoma, rather than something else?

Almost always, the specimen received by a pathologist from someone with suspected RCC is a kidney or part of a kidney. Needle biopsy specimens of a mass in the kidney are unusual but are occasionally taken, e.g. if a neoplasm other than RCC is suspected, such as a lymphoma. Needle biopsy specimens are also taken from masses outside the kidney such as in bone and may show metastatic RCC.

Benign lesions may be confused with RCC. Other malignant neoplasms rarely give problems of discrimination and then only in needle biopsy specimens.

Entities that may be confused with renal cell carcinoma

Particularly in a needle biopsy specimen, adrenal gland, adrenocortical neoplasms and xanthogranulomatous pyelonephritis may resemble clear-cell RCC. In cases of doubt, immunohistology is helpful and will show cytokeratins and epithelial membrane antigen in RCC but not in the other tissues.

There are supposedly benign neoplasms of the kidney, namely papillary adenoma, metanephric adenoma and adenofibroma, and oncocytoma. The distinction between papillary adenoma and papillary carcinoma is currently unsatisfactory because it is based on the size of the neoplasm and some so-called adenomas could be small carcinomas. A papillary neoplasm no more than 5 mm in diameter is considered to be an adenoma (Grignon and Eble 1998). Metanephric adenoma and adenofibroma are rare (Davis et al. 1995; Grignon and Eble 1998). Oncocytoma is common, often has a distinctive brown colour and a central white area, and consists of uniform eosinophilic cells that do not express vimentin on immunohistological study, unlike many RCCs.

What type of renal cell carcinoma is it?

Many elaborate schemes of classification of RCC have been described, mostly of little practical use. Any scheme of value should be shown to be consistent between pathologists, to be applicable in everyday practice and to be related to prognosis. A current classification was suggested apparently independently by two groups in 1997, although three pathologists were in both groups and the reports are similar. This classification is useful in everyday practice because it relies on morphological appearances, even though it was based on cytogenetic findings that are not yet in common use.

Classification of renal cell carcinoma (Kovacs et al. 1997; Storkel et al. 1997)

- Most are common or conventional RCCs, typically clear cell.
- Papillary RCCs were a single group in the original schemes but are now considered to be of two types. One has papillae lined by small cells, often basophilic, and the other has papillae lined by large eosinophilic cells. These are sometimes called type 1 and type 2, respectively, although descriptive names are better than numbers in identification of entities (Delahunt and Eble 1997).
- Chromophobe RCC and collecting duct carcinoma of the kidney are rare but distinctive.
- Unclassified RCC is an unsatisfactory term that may have to be used when no other seems appropriate.
- Sarcomatoid change is seen in all types of RCC and is not considered a separate type of carcinoma in this classification.

Although this classification does not mention neuroendocrine neoplasms of the kidney, these are sometimes included in lists of renal cell neoplasms (Eble and Young 2000).

Value of classification of renal cell carcinoma

Evidence that this scheme was of value was given by two studies with several common authors (Moch et al. 2000; De Peralta-Venturina et al. 2001). These showed that RCCs with sarcomatoid change had a worse prognosis than those without this change, irrespective of the underlying type of carcinoma, that chromophobe renal cell carcinoma had a better prognosis than conventional clear cell carcinoma, and that papillary carcinoma with small cells, so-called type 1, had a better prognosis than papillary carcinoma with large cells, so-called type 2.

What features are present of relevance to prognosis?

The most important prognostic feature in RCC is the extent of spread, i.e. the stage. RCC is usually detected late in its course, and most carcinomas are large and have spread into veins and outside the kidney at diagnosis.

Although various schemes of grading have been described, these have been shown to be poorly reproducible between pathologists (Lanigan et al. 1994). This finding suggests that caution should be used in interpretation of studies that claim that grading of renal cell carcinoma is valuable. The simplest scheme of grading uses only three grades – well differentiated, moderately differentiated and poorly differentiated – and has the least poor reproducibility. For this reason, if grading is considered necessary, this scheme should be used, although there is doubt whether grading is relevant to prognosis (Goldstein 1999; Montironi et al. 1999).

The pathologist should provide information from which the stage can be determined by someone who is aware of all relevant facts. Often the pathologist is not informed of facts such as presentation with a distant metastasis, and the stage given by a pathologist on a nephrectomy specimen would be wrong. The most widespread staging system is the TNM one, although there are others (Montironi et al. 1999).

Features required for TNM staging (Guinan et al. 1997)

The TNM classification does not include the type or grade of RCC. This scheme also makes no mention of multiple or bilateral carcinomas, which are often found, e.g. in von Hippel–Lindau syndrome or acquired cystic disease of the kidney.

The size of the carcinoma is important, provided that there is no evidence of spread into veins or outside the kidney. A carcinoma no more than 7 cm in diameter is called T1 and one over this size is called T2. Spread into major veins or outside the kidney is called T3. Spread into the ipsilateral adrenal gland is called T3a, provided that this is by direct invasion. This is unusual because RCC more often reaches the adrenal gland by invasion of the adrenal vein. Whether this should be called T3a, T3b or M1 is not made clear. Spread into perinephric or peripelvic fat is also called T3a, provided that this is not through the peritoneal lining or into adjacent organs, when this becomes T4, or spread beyond Gerota's fascia. Gerota's fascia is largely a theoretical concept for pathologists and this extent of spread can be determined only if there is direct infiltration of carcinoma into structures adjacent to the kidney, other than the adrenal gland. These structures include liver, bowel, peritoneal lining and abdominal muscles. Assessment of spread into perinephric fat requires appropriate sampling of the surface of a carcinoma and spread means infiltration of fat, not just bulging of the surface of the carcinoma (Montironi et al. 1999). Invasion of the renal pelvis has no prognostic significance (Montironi et al. 1999).

Extension into major renal veins or the inferior vena cava below the diaphragm is called T3b, and extension into the inferior vena cava above the diaphragm is called T3c. The problems here are that, although spread into the main renal vein and inferior vena cava is easy to determine, the pathologist cannot usually say how far up the cava the carcinoma extends, and the definition of major renal veins is vague. These are said to be segmental veins with muscle in their wall. Direct invasion of the wall of the cava is under consideration as an important feature but this is usually not easy for a pathologist to determine, first because only material from the lumen may be received and second because organising thrombus usually obscures the planes between the carcinoma and the original caval wall.

Regional lymph nodes, namely renal hilar, para-aortic and paracaval, are not always received with nephrectomy specimens and the pathologist should report whether there are any lymph nodes and how many there are. Metastasis in one lymph node is called N1 and metastasis in more than one is called N2. With a nephrectomy specimen, the pathologist does not often receive specimens that give evidence of distant metastasis, called M1, but perhaps the most common of these specimens is the contralateral adrenal gland.

Additional information that a pathologist can give on a partial nephrectomy specimen for RCC is the completeness of local resection, i.e. whether the carcinoma contacts the surgical plane of resection through the kidney.

Summary of TNM staging

- Stage 1 corresponds with T1, i.e. a carcinoma ≤ 7 cm in diameter without spread into major veins or outside the kidney.
- Stage 2 corresponds with T2, a carcinoma > 7 cm diameter, but otherwise similar to stage 1.
- Stage 3 means spread into veins, T3b or T3c, and/or into the adrenal gland or perinephric fat, T3a, and/or into one lymph node, N1.
- Stage 4 means spread into adjacent organs other than adrenal gland, T4, and/or into more than one lymph node, N2, and/or into a distant organ, M1.

Most RCCs are at least stage 3 at presentation. Of the last 200 consecutive nephrectomy specimens for RCC seen by the author, 52 were at least stage 1, 14 at least stage 2, 103 at least stage 3 and 31 stage 4.

Conclusions

Pathologists give the diagnosis of RCC. They also determine the type of carcinoma, although this is relatively unimportant, because sarcomatoid differentiation is probably the only common histological change in an RCC of major prognostic significance. Apart from determination of the diagnosis, the other main contribution of pathologists is to investigate and report features relevant to the prognosis, particularly the extent of spread. These are size of the carcinoma, invasion of veins, and infiltration of fat, adrenal gland and other structures outside the kidney. Pathologists are also of great importance in research into the understanding of RCC.

References

Davis CJ, Barton JH, Sesterhenn IA, Mostofi FK (1995) Metanephric adenoma: clinicopathological study of fifty patients. *American Journal of Surgical Pathology* **19**: 1101–1114.

Delahunt B, Eble JN (1997) Papillary renal cell carcinoma: a clinicopathologic and immunohistochemical study of 105 tumors. *Modern Pathology* **10**: 537–544.

De Peralta-Venturina M, Moch H, Amin M et al. (2001) Sarcomatoid differentiation in renal cell carcinoma: a study of 101 cases. *American Journal of Surgical Pathology* **25**: 275–284.

Eble JN, Young RH (2000) Tumors of the urinary tract. In: Fletcher CDM (ed), *Diagnostic Histopathology of Tumors*, 2nd edn. London: Churchill Livingstone, pp 475–493.

Goldstein NS (1999) Grading of renal cell carcinoma. *Urologic Clinics of North America* **26**: 637–642.

Grignon DJ, Eble JN (1998) Papillary and metanephric adenomas of the kidney. *Seminars in Diagnostic Pathology* **15**: 41–53.

Guinan P, Sobin LH, Algaba F et al. (1997) TNM staging of renal cell carcinoma. *Cancer* **80**: 992–993.

Kovacs G, Akhtar M, Beckwith BJ et al. (1997) The Heidelberg classification of renal cell tumours. *Journal of Pathology* **183**: 131–133.

Lanigan D, Conroy R, Barry-Walsh C et al. (1994) A comparative analysis of grading systems in renal adenocarcinoma. *Histopathology* **24**: 473–476.

Moch H, Gasser T, Amin MB et al. (2000) Prognostic utility of the recently recommended histologic classification and revised TNM staging system of renal cell carcinoma: a Swiss experience with 588 tumors. *Cancer* **89**: 604–614.

Montironi R, Mikuz G, Algaba F et al. (1999) Epithelial tumours of the adult kidney. *Virchows Archiv* **434**: 281–290.

Storkel S, Eble JN, Adlakha K et al. (1997) Classification of renal cell carcinoma. *Cancer* **80**: 987–989.

Chapter 5

Defining the place of diagnostic imaging in renal cell carcinoma

Julian E Kabala

Diagnostic imaging may be considered in four overlapping categories: detection, diagnosis, staging and follow-up. There is considerable controversy and uncertainty in each of these areas, which is likely to remain the case for some time as imaging techniques are further refined.

Detection of renal cell carcinoma

The detection of renal cell carcinoma (RCC) generally occurs in four situations: haematuria, incidental finding, signs and symptoms of advanced disease, or while screening high-risk patients.

The screening group although interesting is numerically small. The best defined are patients with von Hippel–Lindau disease. Intra-abdominal malignancy, particularly RCC, is one of the most common causes of mortality in this group of patients. Tumours may be multiple and early diagnosis is important so that nephron-sparing surgery may be offered. Although ultrasonography and magnetic resonance imaging (MRI) have the advantage of avoidance of radiation and intravenous contrast, the presence of multiple renal cysts may conceal small early tumours. As this condition is relatively rare, imaging studies have included only small numbers but, once multiple renal cysts appear, computed tomography (CT) appears to be the best screening modality (Choyke et al. 1990).

Advanced disease refers to patients presenting with any of the numerous symptoms of locally advanced or metastatic RCC. Again this is an interesting but (fortunately) relatively small group. A wide range of signs and symptoms has been described relating to the bulk of the tumour and the effect of metastatic disease, and include fever, malaise, weight loss, jaundice, convulsions, bone pain, anaemia, etc. Once the patient has presented, detection is not particularly a problem (provided the possibility is considered). The primary tumour is usually easily demonstrated with ultrasonography and where appropriate the extent is demonstrated with CT.

Incidentally discovered RCC has become a substantial group in recent years, constituting up to 50% in some series (Dhote et al. 2000). Clearly, this is not really a problem of detection but of diagnosis, determining the nature of the (often small) detected lesion.

From the point of view of detection the single most important group is the assessment of haematuria. Traditionally the gold standard investigation was the intravenous urogram (IVU – Figure 5.1) which remains a useful modality (Webb 1997). Once a mass is detected on IVU, its solid nature is confirmed with ultrasonography (Figure 5.2). More recently, it has been argued that ultrasonography and cystocopy alone are sufficient to investigate haematuria. The advantages are: the avoidance of radiation and the risk of intravenous contrast, and the relatively good availability and speed of the procedure. This availability has been increased by the recent practice of increasingly delegating routine ultrasonographic examinations to trained radiographers. There is therefore a strong current in favour of investigating these patients with ultrasonography alone and many institutions have adopted this pragmatic protocol.

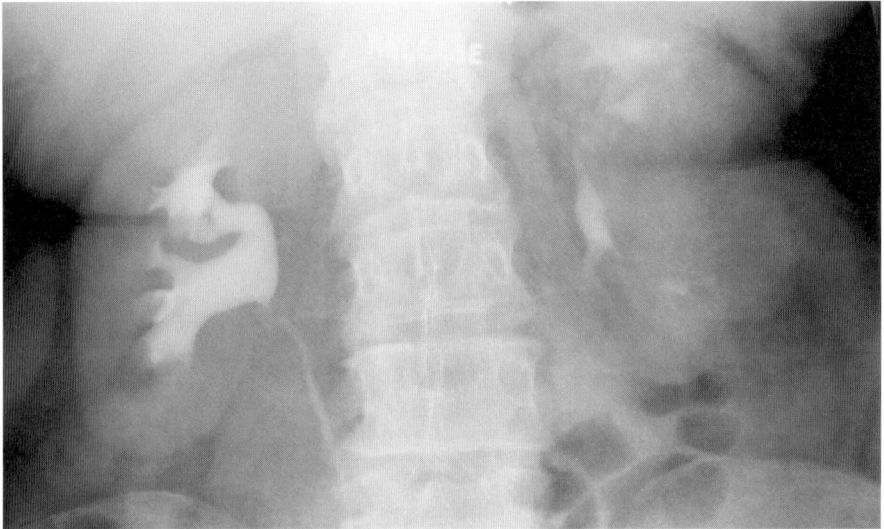

Figure 5.1 Intravenous urogram showing a large left renal mass (subsequently shown to be a renal cell carcinoma) distorting the calyces.

Ultrasonography is sensitive for the detection of masses and appears superior to IVU especially when the masses are small. Warshauer et al. (1988) compared optimal IVU (with tomography) with ultrasonography in 204 patients with renal masses, CT being used as the gold standard. IVU detected only 21% of masses between 1 and 2 cm in diameter and 10% < 1 cm diameter (corresponding figures for ultrasonography being 60% and 26%). Ultrasonography detected three times as many masses with a diameter < 2 cm. It is unlikely that IVU technique has improved significantly since 1988, but ultrasonography undoubtedly has, which suggests its superiority will have increased. A more recent larger study, however, casts doubt on this extrapolation.

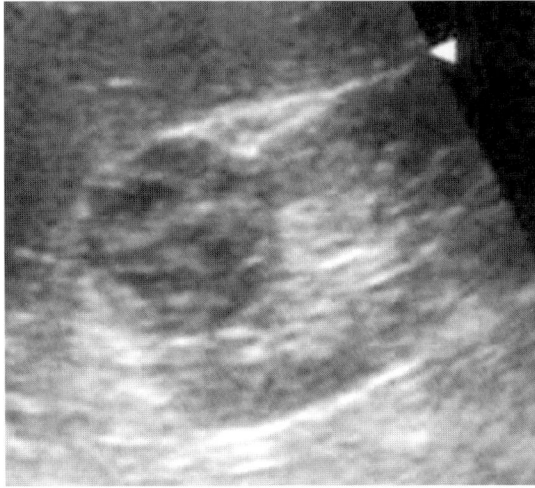

Figure 5.2 Renal ultrasonography demonstrating a small renal cell carcinoma appearing as a slightly heterogeneous mass of predominantly intermediate echogenicity.

Khadra et al. (2000) investigated 1930 patients attending a haematuria clinic using both IVU and ultrasonography; 14 patients were found to have upper tract tumours (12 of them RCC), demonstrating how relatively uncommon upper tract tumours are compared with the number of patients presenting with haematuria. There was a remarkable symmetry to the results in that ultrasonography or IVU alone detected eight tumours but each failed to detect tumours in six cases. All patients without a diagnosis were followed up for a minimum of 2.5 years and none of them demonstrated subsequent tumour development. The conclusion from this data was that both IVU and ultrasonography should be performed on all patients with haematuria, and that this combination will detect all clinically significant upper tract tumours.

The logistics of this suggestion are worth considering. Some studies have found an incidence of microscopic haematuria of up to 38% in a healthy population (Froom et al. 1984), although a figure of around 2.5% of the adult population may be more realistic (Ritchie et al. 1986). This would lead to 10^6 ultrasonographic and IVU studies perhaps annually for this indication alone. This is a considerable commitment of resources as well as an enormous radiation burden (each IVU representing 2.5 mSv or 14 months of background radiation – Royal College of Radiologists 1998) to the population and potentially between 4000 and 40 000 severe reactions to intravenous contrast medium (Thomsen and Morcos 2000).

The incidence of upper tract tumours in patients with haematuria is low (< 1%) and the incidence of patients in whom no diagnosis is made is high (> 50% in macroscopic haematuria and > 70% in microscopic haematuria – Khadra et al. 2000). It has therefore been recommended that initially ultrasonography alone should be used in microscopic haematuria (Dalla Palma 2001), further investigation being indicated only if there is persistence or recurrence. This rests on the (reasonable) assumption that, where a small upper tract urothelial tumour is not shown on initial ultrasonography, it is unlikely to progress significantly in the short period of time before further investigation is arranged. In macroscopic haematuria, the same protocol can be defended although a substantial cohort of radiologists might prefer to use both ultrasonography and IVU at the outset in this group.

Where there is recurrent or persistent haematuria and no cause has been identified on initial investigation, an occult upper tract malignancy is unlikely to be present. In this group repeating the ultrasonography and/or IVU after a period of surveillance (3–6 months) is simple and prudent but only uncommonly reveals a diagnosis. Careful CT with contrast is more sensitive for small upper tract masses, but the yield is low and the radiation burden (10 mSv or 4.5 years of background radiation) and potential contrast sensitivity risk must be considered. Currently, it is unlikely to be used for more than occasional selected cases. MRI does not have the radiation or contrast hazards of CT, but still does not match its sensitivity (McClennan and Deyoe 1994), especially with recent technical advances in the field of CT (spiral and multislice).

With improvements in CT scanners and the reduction in scan times, it has become possible to obtain images during different phases of renal enhancement. The normal renal parenchyma is of intermediate density, measuring between 30 and 60 Hounsfield units (HU). Following intravenous contrast the cortex enhances more rapidly than the medulla, appearing more dense from around 20–60 s when there is maximum corticomedullary differentiation (corticomedullary phase). Around 60–180 s the renal parenchyma becomes homogeneously high density – around 80–120 HU (nephrographic phase). Routine enhanced CT is generally performed in the corticomedullary phase, which is valuable for assessing lesion vascularity (Figure 5.3) and demonstrating normal renal architecture; this is especially valuable in differentiating normal renal tissue (e.g. areas of hypertrophy, prominent column of Bertin, etc.) from pathological masses. However, different lesions have different conspicuity in the corticomedullary and nephrogenic phases. Some highly vascular lesions may be harder to see in the nephrographic phase (Figure 5.4). More often, small lesions, especially when poorly vascular, are better seen in the nephrographic phase (Figure 5.5; Szolar et al. 1997). Despite this, it does not seem currently that the excess radiation and time on the scanner justify performing corticomedullary and nephrogenic phase imaging (multiphase scanning) routinely (Urban 1997).

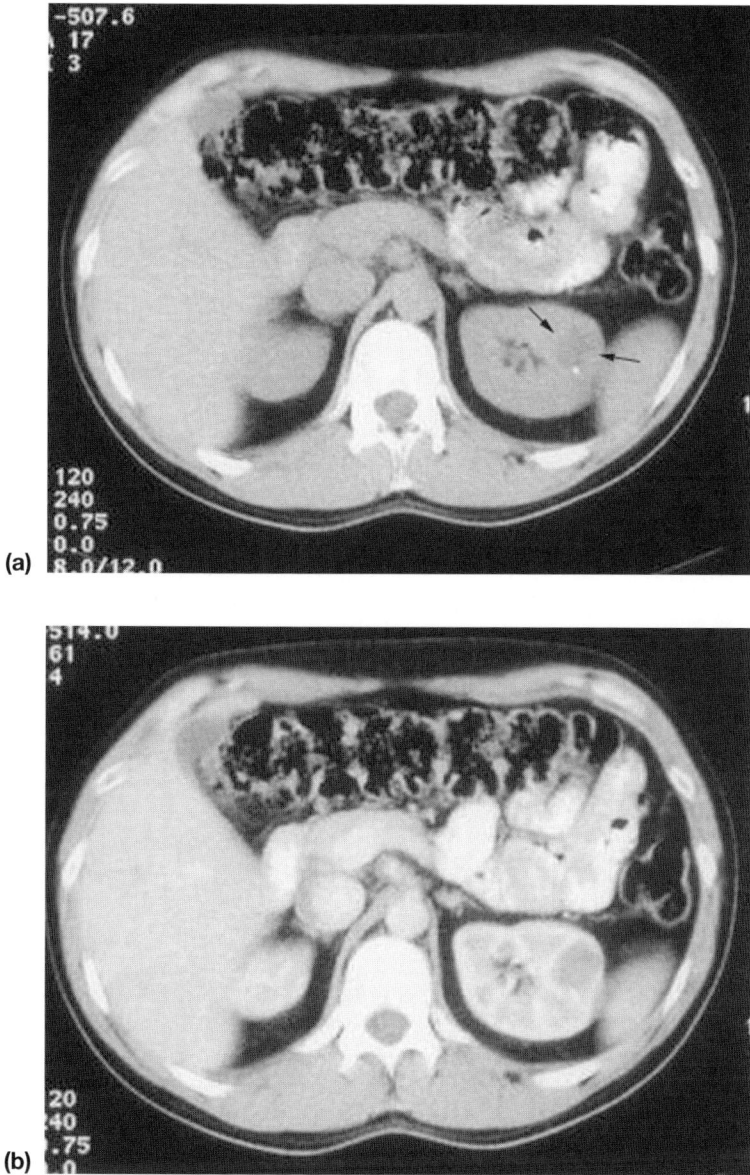

Figure 5.3 Small, relatively poorly vascular renal cell carcinoma demonstrated on computed tomography (CT). (a) The unenhanced images show a slightly ill-defined mass (arrows) with a small focus of calcification lying posteriorly in the left kidney. (b) Scanning in the corticomedullary phase shows the mass to have poor enhancement. Good demonstration of the normal corticomedullary architecture is present.

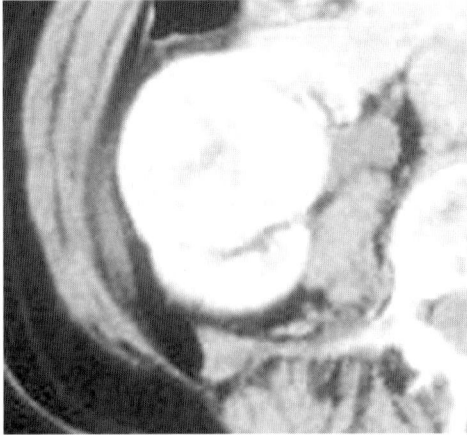

Figure 5.4 Large right renal neoplasm (oncocytoma) showing intense enhancement. Scanning has been performed during the nephrographic phase and the normal renal parenchyma shows a homogeneous high density without any corticomedullary differentiation visible. The tumour is of virtually identical density to normal renal tissue and is mainly identified by virtue of its mass effect.

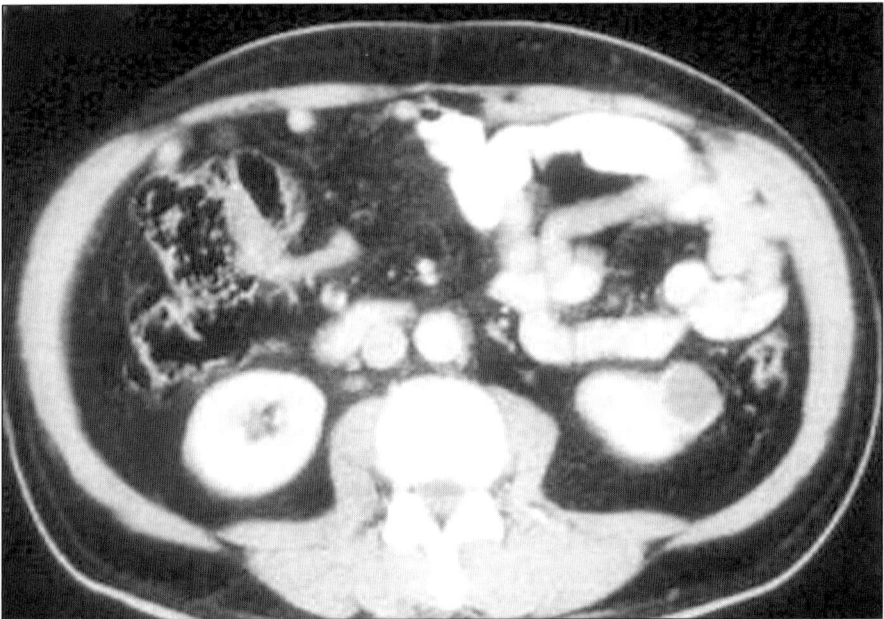

Figure 5.5 Enhanced CT scan showing a classic, non-enhancing, well-defined left renal cyst.

Diagnosis

Having detected a suspicious lesion the next consideration is how accurately the radiologist can predict its nature. A mass may be detected on IVU, but another modality is required to determine its nature. Most patients will therefore undergo ultrasonography and have one of three appearances. The vast majority of masses will be securely categorised as simple cysts on the basis of reliable ultrasonic features. A simple cyst is well defined, homogeneous and echo free, with distal acoustic enhancement and no appreciable wall thickness (Figure 5.6). CT (see Figure 5.5) and MRI (Figure 5.7) show analogous features, with the important addition of complete absence of enhancement with intravenous contrast.

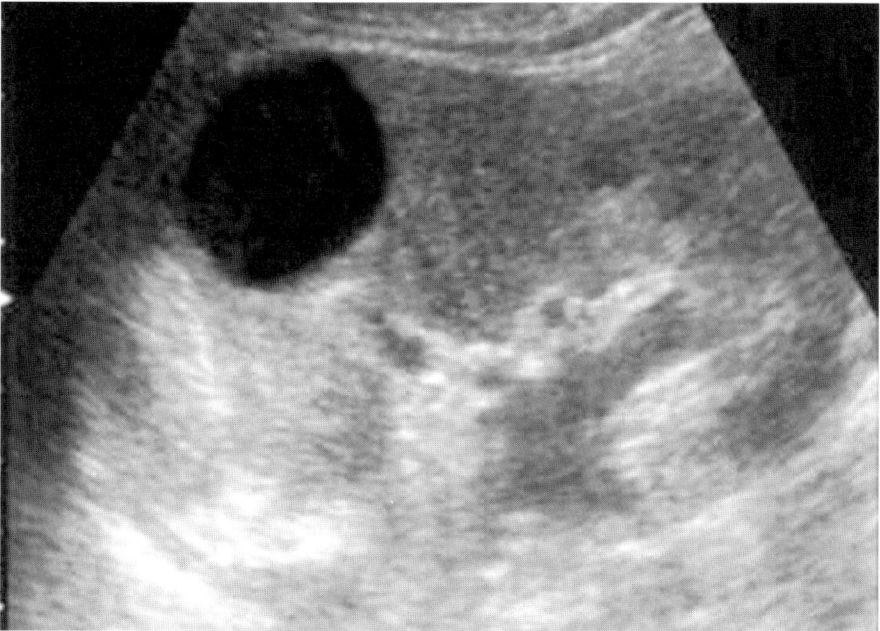

Figure 5.6 Renal ultrasonogram showing a typical well-defined, echo-free cyst with distal acoustic enhancement (note the divergent echogenic area immediately below the cyst).

A significant minority of masses are predominantly solid, of which around 80–85% are RCCs (Fowler and Reznek 2001). The remaining renal masses are indeterminate, being neither an obvious benign cyst nor an obvious RCC. These require further investigation with CT or MRI and include cystic lesions, solid lesions not typical of RCC and small lesions.

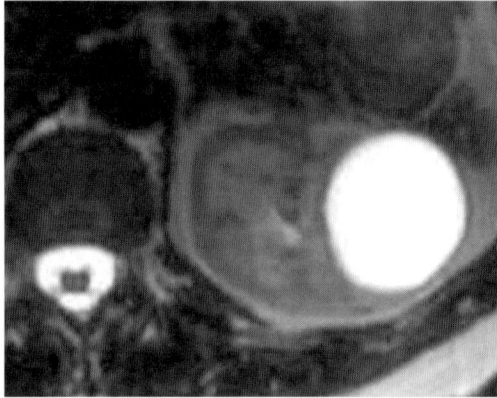

Figure 5.7 Magnetic resonance image of the left kidney (T2-weighted image) showing a classic simple cyst with signal intensity similar to water (compare with the cerebrospinal fluid) and no appreciable wall thickness.

Cystic lesions

Cystic lesions have been classified into four categories on radiological criteria (Bosniak 1986; Table 5.1) to allow some statement about their malignant potential to be made. The original description was of the features seen on CT (Figure 5.8) and this still remains the most reliable way to assess indeterminate lesions (Patel 1999). Similar features, however, can be identified on ultrasonography and MRI. Category I corresponds to a simple cyst, as described above, with a well-defined thin wall and homogeneous water density contents that are not enhanced. Category II cysts may show a few thin (1 mm) septa and fine peripheral calcification. The density on CT may be increased, presumed to result from previous infection or haemorrhage. A well-defined homogeneously dense lesion may represent either a category II cyst or a solid neoplasm. The crucial differentiation between the two rests on a virtually complete lack of enhancement with intravenous contrast in the case of a cyst (rise in density on CT of ≤ 10 HU) compared with demonstrable enhancement in the case of a neoplasm (Macari and Bosniak 1999). Category III cysts include dense and/or thick

Table 5.1 Bosniak classification and probability of malignancy

Stage	Malignancy
I	Simple cyst (0%)
II	Fine septa and/or peripheral calcification ± homogeneous density increase (30%)
III	Thick septa and/or calcification (60%)
IV	Solid areas of enhancement (90%)

From Bosniak (1986) and Koga (2000).

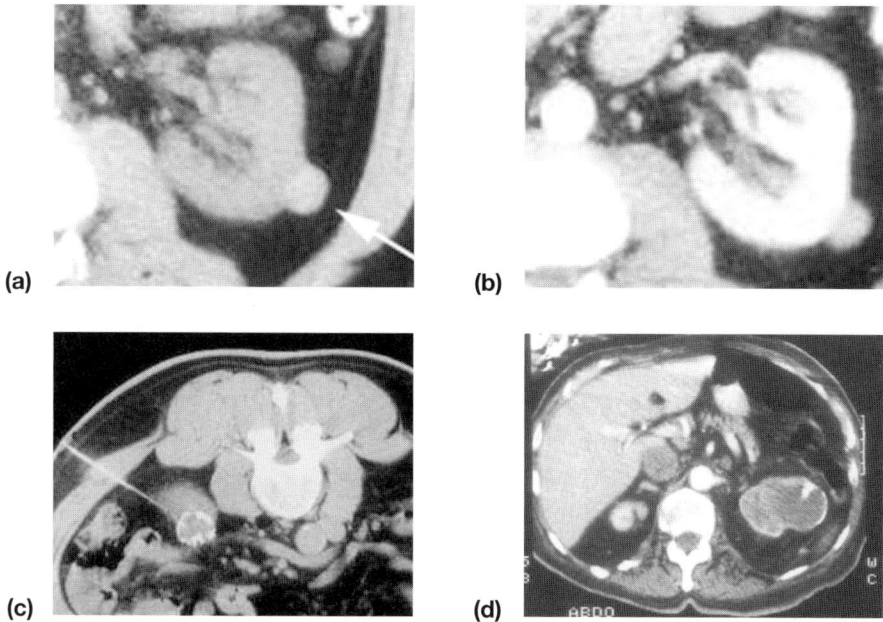

Figure 5.8 CT scan of cystic lesions. (a) A high-density cyst (arrow) with complete lack of enhancement is regarded as (b) a Bosniak type II cyst (following intravenous contrast). (c) Dense calcification is a feature of type III cysts (imaged during CT-guided aspiration). (d) Solid areas of enhancement indicate a type IV cyst (note also the prominent area of calcification).

areas of calcification and multiple, irregular or thickened (> 1 mm) septa. Category IV cysts show solid areas of enhancement and irregular thickened walls and septa that may also enhance.

The usefulness of this classification is that the higher the category the more likely the lesion is to represent a renal malignancy. Approximately 90% of category IV lesions and 60% of category III lesions are malignant (Koga et al. 2000). Both these categories are therefore best treated with surgical excision (category III justifying nephron-sparing surgery). In category II the risk of malignancy is sufficiently low to allow a period of observation with a repeat scan in 6 months. However, differentiation between category II and III is often difficult and subjective, and the category should be reviewed every time imaging is performed. The usefulness of image-guided biopsy remains uncertain (Figure 5.8c) because a negative aspirate does not exclude malignancy. However, if the aspirate demonstrates neoplastic cytology, surgery is indicated without the need for a period of surveillance (Brierly et al. 2000).

Solid lesions not typical of RCC

It is generally safest to assume that a solid renal mass is a RCC and should be treated with radical or partial nephrectomy. However, imaging features may suggest a different diagnosis.

A centrally placed lesion that is more infiltrative than expansile suggests the presence of a transitional cell carcinoma requiring nephroureterectomy. A well-defined tumour with a central scar may represent an oncocytoma (see Figure 5.4), perhaps better treated with partial nephrectomy. Multiple and/or bilateral renal lesions should prompt a search for features of metastases or lymphoma (Figure 5.9) and may require biopsy. Other rare malignancies are encountered on occasion. Renal sarcoma is usually non-specific in appearance, but has a tendency to appear as subcapsular malignant nodules. The presence of fat is virtually pathognomonic of angiomyolipoma, even when only a very small amount is present.

Small lesions

As the quality of scanning equipment improves and the general population is examined more often, there has been an increase in the incidental discovery of small asymptomatic renal masses (Bosniak 1991). This is likely to continue, e.g. as spiral CT becomes more widely used in the investigation of renal colic.

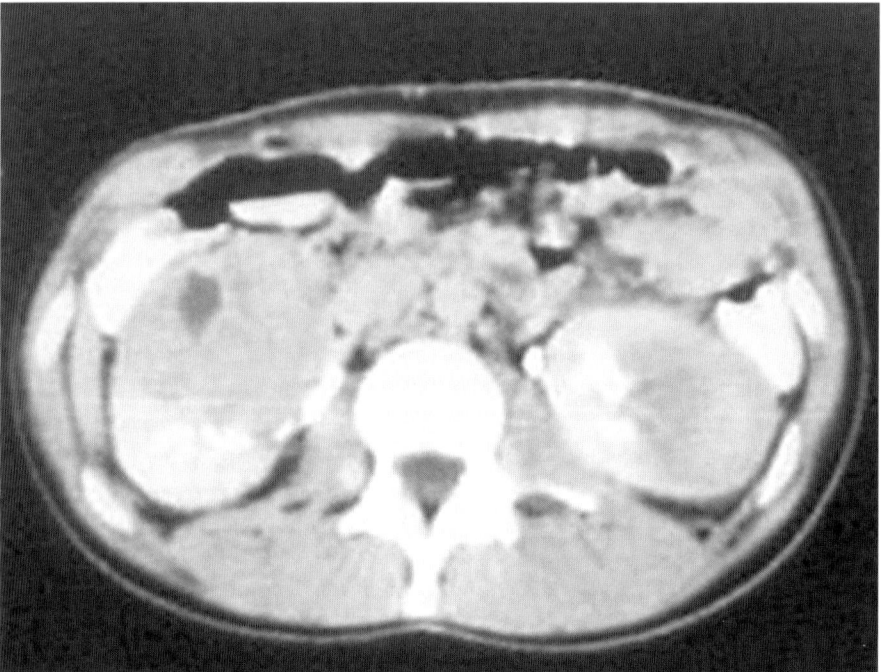

Figure 5.9 CT scan demonstrating large, bilateral, well-defined, predominantly homogeneous deposits of lymphoma.

Lesions that are 1.5–3.0 cm in diameter can usually be adequately categorised as simple cysts, probable RCCs or indeterminate lesions to be considered as above. Very small lesions (< 1.5 cm) may be difficult to categorise, especially if there is an equivocal lesion on CT and the patient's build does not permit adequate visualisation with ultrasonography.

In these circumstances, it would seem reasonable to repeat the imaging after 6 months and then yearly. Small lesions without significant demonstrable increase in size are unlikely to represent aggressive tumours (Birnbaum et al. 1990). If the lesion grows to > 2 cm diameter, then removal, probably with a partial nephrectomy, would be appropriate (Fowler and Reznek 2001).

Staging

Once the diagnosis has been made the tumour requires staging. It is useful for the radiologist to be familiar with the staging systems in current use (TNM and Robson – Table 5.2) which formalises the information the surgeon requires to plan appropriate treatment (Robson et al. 1969, Reznek 1998). Imaging should describe tumour invasion through the renal capsule, venous invasion, lymph node involvement and extension into adjacent organs.

CT and MRI both have a reported staging accuracy of 90% or more (Johnson et al. 1986; Kabala et al. 1991). However, the error rate for assessing perinephric invasion (transcapsular extension) has been reported to be as high as 50% (Levine 1995). Tumours that are confined by the renal capsule should show a normal perinephric space (Figure 5.10). Features of extension through the renal capsule include bulk tumour outside the capsule, ill-defined marginal tumours, perinephric stranding and fascial thickening (Figure 5.11). However, some of these features may also occur in confined tumours as a result of adjacent reactive inflammatory change, oedema or

Table 5.2 Combined Robson and TNM staging system for renal cell carcinoma

Robson	TNM
I (limited by the renal capsule)	T1 ($\leq$ 7.0 cm)
II (perinephric extension)	T2 (> 7.0 cm)
IIIa (tumour invasion into renal vein or IVC)	T3a (perinephric extension)
IIIb (tumour involvement of regional lymph nodes)	T3b (extension into renal vein or infradiaphragmatic IVC)
IIIc (venous and lymph node invasion)	T3c (extension into the supradiaphragmatic IVC)
IV (invasion of adjacent viscera or distant metastases)	T4 (tumour invades beyond Gerota's fascia)

IVC, inferior vena cava.

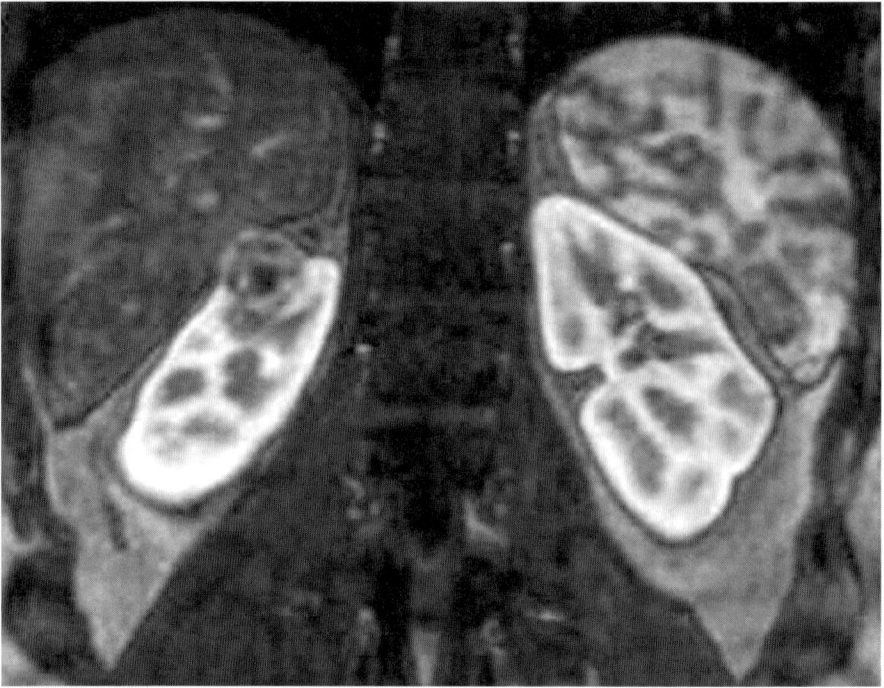

Figure 5.10 Coronal MRI (FLASH three-dimensional) showing a small renal cell carcinoma confined to the kidney, the adjacent perinephric space being entirely normal.

collateral blood supply. Conventional treatment with radical nephrectomy is offered regardless of extension through the renal capsule, and this degree of local spread makes little difference to the prognosis. Currently, however, nephron-sparing surgery (partial nephrectomy) is increasingly being offered if the tumour is confined by the capsule. When this procedure is contemplated accurate local staging becomes much more important. A recent series (Pretorius et al. 1999), specifically looking at assessment for partial nephrectomy with MRI before and after intravenous gadolinium enhancement, demonstrated extremely high accuracy in the differentiation of confined tumours from those showing extension through the capsule. Tumour confined to the kidney was correctly predicted in 38 of 39 cases whereas tumour extension outside the capsule was correctly predicted in two of three cases. This, however, was clearly a series of small lesions already selected for partial nephrectomy, in which the vast majority were predictably confined tumours.

The overall accuracy for staging lymph node involvement with CT and MRI is around 83–89% (Nikken and Krestin 2000; Rankin et al. 2000). Detection of involved lymph nodes, however, depends on nodal enlargement > 1 cm diameter (Figure 5.12). Unfortunately, this leads to a substantial number of false positives

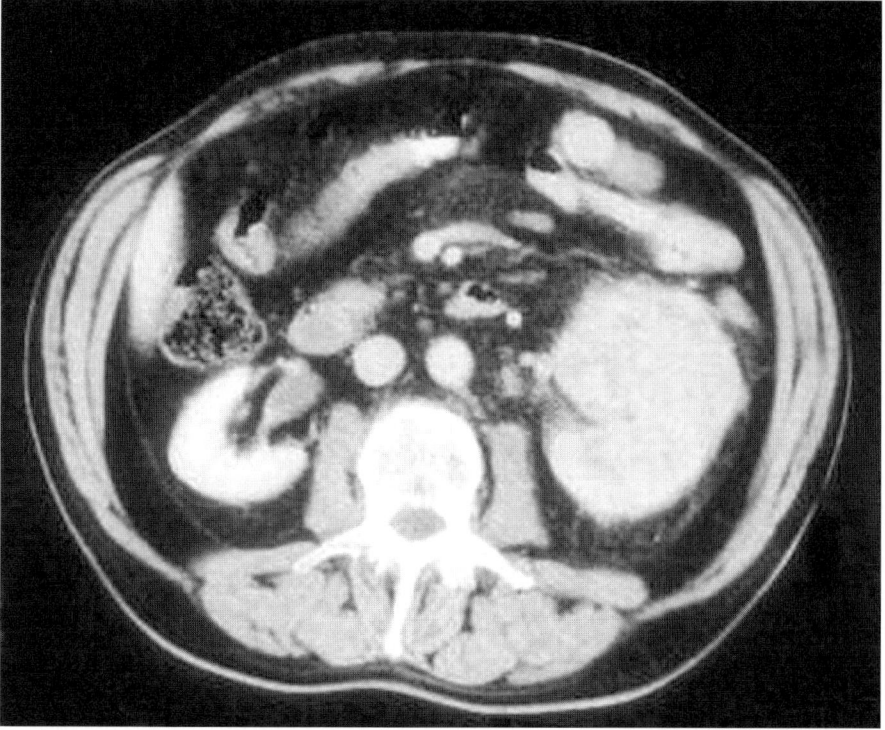

Figure 5.11 CT scan showing a large left-sided renal cell carcinoma with extension into the perinephric space.

resulting from reactive inflammatory hyperplasia, up to 43% in some studies (Studer et al. 1990). Enlargement to > 2 cm diameter is almost always caused by metastases. False negatives are encountered less often, with microscopic metastases in the absence of lymph node enlargement being much less common.

CT and MRI reliably demonstrate venous invasion with an accuracy of 80–90% for invasion into the renal vein and in excess of 95% for the inferior vena cava (Welch and LeRoy 1997; Nikken et el 2000). There is little difference between the modalities and, in routine practice, the choice will reflect local experience and the availability of modern scanners. The full extent of tumour is usually well demonstrated (Figure 5.13) and once tumour extends into the inferior vena cava its direction of spread is usually superiorly with the flow of blood, occasionally as far as the right atrium.

CT and MRI are generally reliable for the demonstration of tumour invasion into adjacent organs (Figure 5.14). The organs involved are predictable from the relationships of the kidneys, and include posterior extension into the psoas muscle and quadratus lumborum, superiorly into the adrenal glands, laterally into the abdominal wall, posterosuperiorly into the diaphragm, and anteriorly into the colon, liver and duodenum

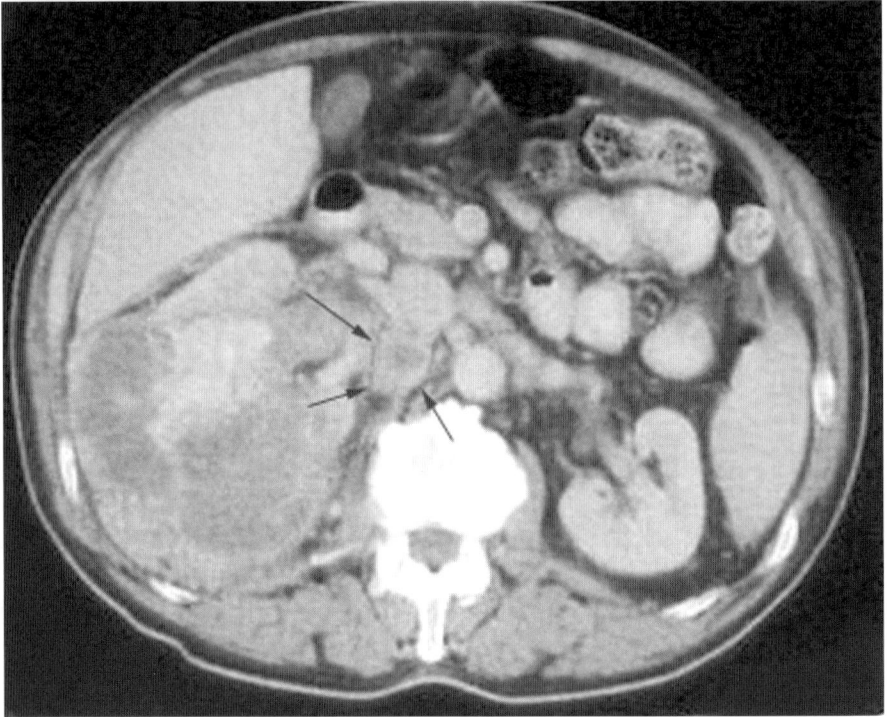

Figure 5.12 CT scan showing a large right-sided renal cell carcinoma with adjacent lymph node metastasis (arrows).

(on the right) and pancreas, jejunum, stomach and spleen (on the left). Loss of the fat line between the tumour and adjacent structure on CT or MRI is common, and in itself does not necessarily indicate invasion, the diagnosis requiring the demonstration of density/signal change and/or enlargement (Reznek 1998).

In addition to accurate staging, partial nephrectomy requires optimal demonstration of the tumour location within the kidney and the relationship of the tumour to the blood supply with any variants of the renal arteries. Good quality CT or MRI with a vascular programme is reliable for these purposes and formal angiography is rarely indicated (Coll et al. 1999). Spiral CT with a contrast infusion and relatively narrow collimation and image reconstruction (e.g. 3 mm and 1.5 mm respectively; pitch of 1–1.6) is suitable for demonstration of the renal arteries and major branches. MR protocols continue to evolve. A FLASH three-dimensional sequence with bolus tracking is illustrated in Figure 5.15.

Follow-up of patients after treatment for RCC varies across different institutions. The simplest protocol includes annual chest radiography and ultrasonography to assess the renal bed (or remnant) and monitor the contralateral kidney for the presumed increased risk of metachronous disease. Annual spiral CT has been advocated

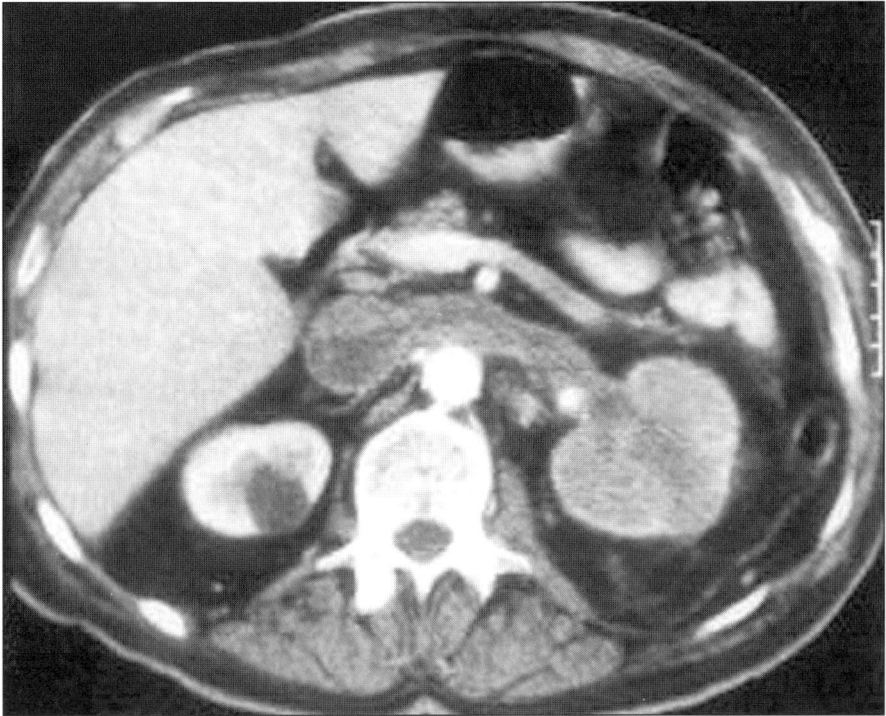

Figure 5.13 CT scan showing a left-sided renal cell carcinoma with gross extension into the renal vein and inferior vena cava. Incidental note is made of a classic right-sided simple renal cyst.

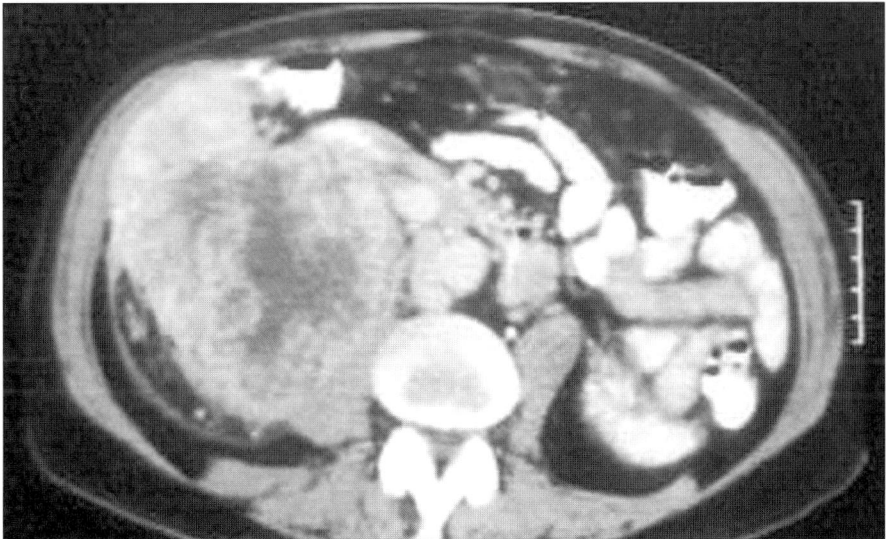

Figure 5.14 CT scan showing a large advanced right-sided renal cell carcinoma with invasion of the perinephric fat, fascia and adjacent abdominal wall.

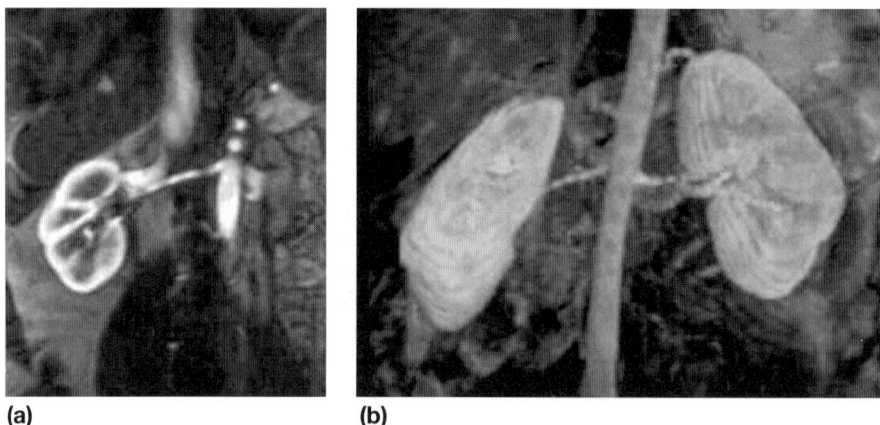

(a)   (b)

Figure 5.15 MRI demonstrating renal vasculature. (a) Oblique coronal image from a FLASH three-dimensional series, showing both the right renal vein (and Inferior vena cava) and the renal artery. (b) Three-dimensional images can be derived from this sequence by a process of maximum intensity projection.

(Rankin et al. 2000), which is undoubtedly more sensitive. The cost in radiation and scanning time, however, requires consideration and arguably this modality should be reserved for patients with a particularly high risk of recurrence such as a strong family history or papillary carcinoma (Turner 2000).

Conclusion

Initial detection of RCC is still predominantly in the context of haematuria with a second sizable group of incidentally discovered tumours. Initial investigation is with ultrasonography and/or IVU, often with ultrasonography alone. Where no diagnosis is made, especially with persistent haematuria, follow-up investigations and/or specialist studies are indicated and may include contrast CT.

Initial lesion categorisation with ultrasonography is likely to be successful in the majority, with others requiring CT, biopsy and/or follow-up to determine their nature. Currently, there is little to choose between CT and MRI for staging tumours, both modalities being generally excellent and adequate also for work-up for partial nephrectomy.

References

Bosniak MA (1986) The current radiological approach to renal cysts. *Radiology* **158**: 1–10.
Bosniak MA (1991) The small (<3cm) renal parenchymal tumour: detection, diagnosis and controversies. *Radiology* **179**: 307–317.
Birnbaum BA, Bosniak MA, Megibow AJ, Lubat E, Gordon RB (1990) Observations on the growth of renal neoplasms. *Radiology* **176**: 695–701.

Brierly RD, Thomas PJ, Harrison NW, Fletcher MS, Nawrocki JD, Ashton-Key RE (2000) Evaluation of fine-needle aspiration cytology for renal masses. *British Journal of Radiology International* **85**: 14–18.

Choyke PL, Filling-Katze MR, Shawker TH et al. (1990) Von Hippel–Lindau disease: Radiologic screening for visceral manifestations. *Radiology* **174**: 815–820.

Coll DM, Uzzo RG, Herts BR, Davros WJ, Wirth SL, Novick AC (1999) 3-dimensional rendered computerized tomography for preoperative evaluation and intraoperative treatment of patients undergoing nephron sparing surgery. *Journal of Urology* **161**: 1097–1102.

Dalla Palma L (2001) What is left of IV urography. *European Radiology* **11**: 931–939.

Dhote R, Pellicer-Coeuret M, Thiounn N, Debre B, Vidal-Trecan GR, (2000) Risk factors for adult renal cell carcinoma: a systematic review and implications for prevention. *British Journal of Urology International* **86**: 20–27.

Fowler C, Reznek R (2001) The indeterminate renal mass. *Imaging* **13**(1): 27–43.

Froom P, Ribak J, Benbassat J (1984) Significance of microhaematuria in young adults. *British Medical Journal* **288**: 20–22.

Johnson CD, Dunnick NR, Cohan RH, Illescas FF (1986) Renal adenocarcinoma: CT staging of 100 tumours. *American Journal of Roentgenology* **148**: 59–63.

Kabala JE, Gillett DA, Persad RA, Penry JB, Gingell, JC, Chadwick D (1991) Magnetic resonance imaging in the staging of renal cell carcinoma. *British Journal of Radiology* **64**: 683–689.

Khadra MH, Pickard RS, Charlton M, Powell PH, Neal DE (2000) A prospective analysis of 1,930 patients with haematuria to evaluate current diagnostic practice. *Journal of Urology* **163**: 524–527.

Koga S, Nishikido M, Inuzuka S et al. (2000) An evaluation of Bosniak's radiological classification of cystic renal masses. *British Journal of Urology International* **86**: 607–609.

Levine E (1995) Renal cell carcinoma: Clinical aspects, imaging diagnosis and staging. *Seminars in Roentgenology* **30**: 128–148.

Macari M, Bosniak MA (1999) Delayed CT to evaluate renal masses incidentally discovered at contrast-enhanced CT: Demonstration of vascularity with de-enhancement. *Radiology* **213**: 674–680.

McClennan BL, Deyoe LA (1994) The imaging evaluation of renal cell carcinoma: diagnosis and staging. *Radiologic Clinics of North America* **32**: 55–70.

Nikken JJ, Krestin GP (2000) Magnetic resonance in the diagnosis of renal masses. *British Journal of Urology* International **86**(suppl 1): 58–69.

Patel U (1999) Small and indeterminate renal masses: characterisation and management. *CME Journal of Radiology* **2**: 47–56.

Pretorius ES, Siegelman ES, Rachmandani P, Cangiano T, Banner MP (1999) Renal neoplasms amenable to partial nephrectomy: MR Imaging. *Radiology* **212**: 28–34.

Rankin SC, Webb JAW, Reznek RH (2000) Spiral computed tomography in the diagnosis of renal masses. *British Journal of Urology International* **86**(suppl 1): 48–57.

Reznek R (1998) Renal tumours. In: *Imaging in Oncology*. Oxford: Isis Medical Media, pp. 191–214.

Ritchie CD, Bevan EA, Collier SJ (1986) Importance of occult haematuria found at screening. *British Medical Journal* **292**: 681–683.

Robson CJ, Churchill BM, Anderson W (1969) The results of radical nephrectomy for renal cell carcinoma. *Journal of Urology* **101**: 297–301.

Royal College of Radiologists (1998) Making the best use of a department of clinical radiology. London: The Royal College of Radiologists.

Studer UE, Scherz S, Scheidegger J (1990) Enlargement of regional lymph nodes in renal cell carcinoma is often not due to metastases. *Journal of Urology* **144**: 243–245.

Szolar DH, Kammerhuber F, Altzeiber S (1997) Multiphasic helical CT of the kidney: increased conspicuity for detection and characterisation of small (<3cm) renal masses. *Radiology* **202**: 211–217.

Thomsen HS, Morcos SK (2000) Radiographic contrast media. *British Journal of Radiology International* **86**(suppl 1): 1–10.

Turner KJ (2000) Inherited renal cancer. *British Journal of Urology International* **86**: 155–164.

Urban BA (1997) The small renal mass: what is the role of multiphasic helical scanning? *Radiology* **202**: 22–23.

Warshauer DM, McCarthy SM, Street L et al. (1988) Detection of renal masses: sensitivities and specificities of excretory urography/linear tomography, US and CT. *Radiology* **169**: 363–365.

Webb JAW (1997) Imaging in haematuria. *Radiology* **52**: 167–171.

Welch TJ, LeRoy AJ (1997) Helical and electron beam CT scanning in the evaluation of renal vein involvement in patients with renal cell carcinoma. *Journal of Computer Assisted Tomography* **21**: 467–471.

PART 3

Surgical intervention

The evidence for conventional approaches to the management of locoregional renal cell carcinoma

Sarah Richards and Alastair WS Ritchie

There are no meta-analyses and few randomised trials to guide management of localised renal cell carcinoma (RCC). Most evidence in support of treatment comes from observational studies relating the surgical and pathological extent of disease to survival. The only reliable, curative treatment for RCC is surgery resulting in complete surgical excision. Tumour spread is highly resistant to therapy, although a few durable responses have followed immunotherapy. In 2000 better survival rates in patients with RCC using the newly revised 1997 TNM system were demonstrated than had ever been reported previously (Tsui et al. 2000a); these were entirely attributed by the authors to recent advances in diagnosis and treatment of the disease.

Assessment of the clinical evidence for the evolving role of surgery in this disease will always be difficult. This results mainly from the continual evolution in the staging of RCC. The first well-recognised staging system was described in 1958 by Flocks and Kadesky; this was later refined by Robson et al. (1969) who proposed further staging of the tumour according to presence of vascular involvement (Table 6.1). Despite this refinement, the staging system did not correlate well with prognosis. The TNM system (Table 6.2) proved to be a more accurate staging system, but was regarded as too complex until simplified in 1992. Groupings were re-organised into stages according to tumour size, vascular spread, lymph node involvement and distant metastases. For the first time a disease-staging system for RCC was shown to correlate with survival (Hofmockel et al. 1995).

Table 6.1 Original Robson staging compared with 1997 TNM criteria

Stage	TNM equivalent	Comment
I	T1N0M0	Tumour confined to renal parenchyma with renal capsule intact
II	T2N0M0	Tumour invading perirenal fat
III	T3N0–1M0 and T1–2N1M0	Tumour invading renal vein, vena cava and lymph nodes
IV	T4N0–2M0–1 and T1–4N2M0 and T1–4N0–1M1	Tumour with distant metastasis and invading adjacent organs

Table 6.2 TNM classification of renal cell carcinoma (TNM 1997)

T	Primary tumour
TX	Primary tumour cannot be assessed
T0	No evidence of primary tumour
T1	Tumour < 7 cm in greatest dimension, confined to kidney
T2	Tumour > 7 cm in greatest dimension, confined to kidney
T3	Tumour extends into major veins, or invades adrenal or perinephric tissues but not beyond Gerota's fascia
T3a	Tumour invades adrenal gland or perinephric tissues but not beyond Gerota's fascia
T3b	Tumour extends into renal vein or vena cava below diaphragm
T3c	Tumour extends into vena cava above diaphragm
T4	Tumour invades beyond Gerota's fascia
N	Regional lymph nodes
NX	Regional lymph nodes cannot be assessed
N0	No regional lymph node metastasis
N1	Metastasis to a single regional lymph node
N2	Metastasis in more than one regional lymph node
M	Distant metastasis
MX	Distant metastasis cannot be assessed
M0	No distant metastasis
M1	Distant metastasis

Historically speaking, changes in staging systems used by different authors make comparison between published series of various surgical interventions difficult. The first series published in the literature on improved survival rates after simple nephrectomy was started in 1910 (Priestley 1939). Comparison of outcome in studies published over 90 years later is obviously complex. The revised TNM criteria in 1997 reclassified stage I tumours from < 5 cm to < 7 cm in size. In spite of this, survival rates appear to be improving.

Advances in imaging modalities have made initial disease staging and disease follow-up far more accurate. Widespread use of ultrasonography and computed tomography (CT) has resulted in the detection of large numbers of incidental tumours which are generally less advanced and have better survival than symptomatic tumours (Siow et al. 2000).

Despite these variable factors and a healthier population, survival rates appear to be improving (Table 6.3). In this chapter, we have attempted to summarise the evidence base for conventional surgical management of RCC.

Table 6.3 Five-year survival for renal cell carcinoma

Stage	5-year survival rate (%) in				
	1981	1986	1992	1995	2000
I	65	88	73	75	91
II		67	68	63	74
III		40	51	38	67
IV	2	2	20	11	32
Number of patients	506	326	314	2473	643
Authors	McNichols et al. (1981)	Golimbu et al. (1986)	Dinney et al. (1992)	Guinan et al. (1995)	Tsui et al. (2000a)

The natural history of RCC: a baseline for treatment comparison

Renal cell carcinoma is the third most common urological malignancy and affects 3/10 000 Americans per year. UK Cancer Research Campaign data for 1995 reported an incidence of 5250 cases. It is commonly acknowledged as a highly variable and unpredictable disease. It may grow to huge sizes with extensive vascular involvement without metastases or produce distant metastases from a primary tumour of < 2 cm.

Most patients with a symptomatic tumour will die within a year of diagnosis. Riches et al. (1951) reviewed their series and found 3% of patients with 'operable' disease, who had not been treated alive 5 years later.

Approximately 30% of patients will have distant metastases at diagnosis. De Kernion et al. (1978) found that, of these patients, 53% were alive at 6 months whereas only 13% survived for longer than 5 years, even if treated aggressively with nephrectomy and adjuvant therapies.

Other prognostic factors include stage, grade, performance status and mode of presentation (incidental versus symptomatic). Variables may also include primary tumour size. Guinan et al. (1995) found a strong statistical correlation in tumour size with survival, especially in stage II disease. To a lesser degree, cell types with in particular a predominance of clear and granular cells and particular histological patterns correlate with improved survival.

The evidence for simple nephrectomy

Wallcott carried out the first simple nephrectomy described in 1861 for RCC; the preoperative diagnosis was hepatic cyst haemorrhage. The operation involves removal of the kidney from Gerota's fascia, leaving adrenal gland, perirenal fat and lymph nodes *in situ*.

It became the standard operation in the 1900s for RCC. No stage-specific survival rates are available and crude survival rates for stages I–III of disease are quoted by various authors in Table 6.4. These are 13–50% at 5 years and 16–39% at 10 years.

The operative mortality rate was reported as 5% by Skinner et al. (1971) and 4% by Riches et al. (1951), although this rose to 13% in this group if there was renal vein involvement.

Table 6.4 Survival rates following simple nephrectomy: stages I–III – major studies

Study	Number of cases	5-year survival rate (%)	10-year survival rate (%)
Mintz and Gaul (1939)	127	13	Unknown
Priestley and Foot (1939)	392	38	27
Humphreys et al. (1960)	165	35	18
Riches et al. (1951)	940	28	16
Skinner et al. (1971)	93	50	39

The results shown in Table 6.4 were a definite improvement over those quoted by Riches et al. (1951) for 'operable' disease that was not treated – 3% at 5 years. However, without stage-specific survival rates available, no comment can be made on the appropriateness of this procedure in all stages of RCC.

Skinner et al. (1971) retrospectively staged all patients in their series who were treated by simple nephrectomy between 1935 and 1948. The results are shown in Table 6.5. The authors suggested from their study that unexpectedly poor stage II survival rates were the result of incomplete removal of tumour deposit in surrounding perirenal fat. These authors suggested that this particular group of patients might benefit from radical nephrectomy.

Table 6.5 Stage-specific survival rates in patients treated by simple nephrectomy (Skinner et al. 1971)

Stage	5-year survival rate (%)
I	62
II	40
III	54

The evidence for radical nephrectomy

There have been advances in surgical techniques from the 1930s to the 1960s, when simple nephrectomy for RCC was routine. Similarly there have been major advances in the understanding of the pathogenesis of neoplasms. As advances were made, theory dictated that the widest possible surgical excision margin should be achieved.

There are more or less simultaneous reports in the literature describing radical nephrectomy. Mortensen (1948) reported radical nephrectomy by thoracoabdominal incision which also involved removal of the spleen and the tail of the pancreas. Chute et al. (1949) also described radical nephrectomy by the thoracoabdominal approach. The basis for radical nephrectomy involves early ligation of renal vessels and removal of Gerota's fascia and contents, i.e. the whole kidney, adrenal gland and perinephric fat. Many methods to establish access are used and include extraperitoneal flank, thoracoabdominal, lumbar, abdominal transperitoneal and extrapleural approaches.

Little effort was made to corroborate this theory on improved survival with extensive tumour field excision, until an initial report on the results of radical nephrectomy was delivered by Robson at the meeting of the American Urological Association in 1962. He went on to publish the full results of the series in 1969 (Robson et al. 1969). He found that 28% of cases had perinephric fat involvement and 22% had lymph node involvement in pathological specimens. These survival rates were compared by graph in the report by Robson, with four other large series of cases of simple nephrectomy including those by Priestley (1939) and Riches et al. (1951), and a statistical improvement was found in the survival rate. This result was based on figures published for all stages and was not case matched. He reported a 52% 5-year survival rate for the whole series. Robson's very good results may, however, be attributable to extensive patient selection to eliminate patients with metastatic disease. Robson employed lung tomograms and mediastinoscopy techniques that were not routinely used by other authors at the time.

Robson concluded that the success of radical nephrectomy was the result of early ligation of the renal artery and vein, complete removal of the perinephric envelope and surgical extirpation of the lymphatic field. The 'gold standard' operation was born and continued largely unchallenged until recent times.

Similarly, after the initial theory proposed by Skinner et al. (1971) that radical nephrectomy may improve survival in stage II disease, they went on retrospectively to stage and compare disease treated in their series by simple nephrectomy up to 1945 with disease treated by radical nephrectomy up to 1971. Their results showed perinephric fat or regional node involvement in 29% of potentially curable patients Their results are displayed in Table 6.6.

Table 6.6 Survival rates in patients undergoing simple and radical nephrectomy (Skinner et al. 1971)

Stage	5 year survival rate (%) for	
	Simple nephrectomy	*Radical nephrectomy*
I	62	68
II	40	50
III	54	49

They concluded that the results of treatment by radical nephrectomy in stage II disease showed an improvement in survival by 10% at 5 years. However, no significant statistical difference could be demonstrated; their results were also separated by 20 years of surgical experience. Despite this, the authors went on to conclude that the principles of surgery dictate that the best operation in this group of patients should involve removal of Gerota's fascia and contents thereby corroborating Robson's earlier published report.

In 1989, Wood and Herr reviewed these series and stated that the benefit of radical over simple nephrectomy remained undemonstrated. More recently, further retrospective series have been published showing the long-term results of simple and radical nephrectomy. Ramon et al. (1990) reviewed 109 simple and radical nephrectomies performed before 1983. They found a significant statistical difference in 5-year survival rate in stage I disease only – 84% survival for radical nephrectomy versus 72% for simple nephrectomy. Although promising figures were initially received for radical over simple nephrectomy for stages II and III disease, these were found not to be statistically significant once non-cancer deaths were excluded and disease stages were matched.

Modern series of patients having radical nephrectomy (Ljungberg et al. 1998; Tsui et al. 2000a) have shown excellent local disease control with local recurrence rates between 0 and 2%. Ljungberg et al. (1998) reported a surgical complication rate of 3%. Corman et al. (2000) have compared mortality and morbidity from radical and partial nephrectomy in a large series of patients receiving treatment at Veterans Administration hospitals, and have reported an operative mortality rate of 2% and 30-day morbidity rate of 15% for radical nephrectomy (Table 6.7).

Table 6.7 Comparison of mortality and morbidity for radical and partial nephrectomy

	Radical nephrectomy (n = 1291)	Partial nephrectomy (n = 468)
30-day mortality rate (%)	2.0	1.6
30-day morbidity rate (%)	15	16.2

Such results do not exclude possible superiority of less radical procedures but give good data on current survival rates following radical nephrectomy, for comparison with less extensive surgery in the form of laparoscopic nephrectomy or nephron-sparing surgery should these be considered as therapeutic alternatives.

The evidence for lymphadenectomy as a component of radical nephrectomy

Robson et al. (1969) questioned the value of dissection of regional lymph nodes. Indeed, pathological evidence of lymph node-positive disease in RCC appears to result in a striking decrease in survival rate (de Kernion et al. 1978). Golimbu et al.

(1986), in studying prognostic factors in RCC, noted that node-positive disease was an ominous prognostic sign resulting in 5-year survival rates falling from 40% to 17% in stage III disease.

Whether extensive dissection of these retroperitoneal nodes is advantageous in terms of prognosis, survival and local control is debatable. The operation itself is longer and more technically demanding and may therefore be expected to impact on patient morbidity and mortality.

Several studies have attempted to resolve the controversy surrounding the merits of lymphadenectomy but only one of these is a prospective randomised trial.

Those arguing against lymphadenectomy do so for several reasons other than just assuming an increase in patient morbidity. First, they query the advantage of removing nodes other than those at the renal hilum which would be removed at routine radical nephrectomy because the distribution of lymphatic metastases is so poorly understood. Siatoh (1982) described over 1800 postmortem examinations for RCC in which lymph node-positive disease was found in unpredictable sites around the body. Second, it is well known that many patients die of disseminated disease despite initial regional node-negative status and absence of localised disease recurrence; this is attributed to blood-borne rather than lymphatic metastases.

The reported incidence of node-positive disease is hugely variable and adds to confusion over the merits of lymph node dissection (Table 6.8).

Table 6.8 Incidence of lymph node-positive disease in published series

Study	Year	Patient group	Node-positive disease (%)
Robson et al.	1969	All	23
Skinner et al.	1972b	All	6
Guilani et al.	1983	pT1–2	5
		pT3–4	36
Herrlinger et al.	1991	All	15
Giberti et al.	1997	pT1	6
		pT2	5
		pT3	10
Blom et al.	1999	All	3

Behind the decision to perform lymphadenectomy for other solid tumours is the principle that lymphatic metastases follow a predictable and reproducible pattern. However, this has been shown not always to be the case in RCC. In 1935 Parker discovered three principal channels of lymphatic drainage from the kidney: a left lumbar, interaortocaval and lateral caval channels to a relatively constant degree, but a highly variable number of pre- and post-aortic, pre- and postcaval and sacral pathways.

Similarly, the node status does not always accurately reflect the extent of the disease. Zisman et al. (2003) reported that 37% of patients with distant metastases had negative nodes at surgery. This suggests that lymphadenectomy offers modest information as to disease stage.

Two major retrospective series are by Giberti et al. (1997) and Schafhauser et al. (1999); both have concluded that there is marginal improvement in patient survival following retroperitoneal lymph node dissection and radical nephrectomy versus radical nephrectomy alone. Giberti et al. (1997) evaluated 328 patients treated by lymphadenectomy retrospectively. The overall 5-year survival rate for these patients was 50.7% at 5 years. They found that lymph node-positive disease had minor importance as a prognostic factor in these patients – 53.2% of patients with lymph node-positive disease survived 5 years and they attributed this finding to completeness of lymph node dissection. Schaufhauser et al. (1995) retrospectively studied 1035 patients treated by curative intervention; patients treated by radical nephrectomy and lymphadenectomy (group A) were compared with groups undergoing radical nephrectomy with removal of suspected macroscopically involved nodes (group B) and radical nephrectomy alone (group C). A breakdown of these results can be seen in Table 6.9.

Table 6.9 Benefits of lymphadenectomy

Group	No. of patients*	Mean age (years)	Median no. of nodes involved	Long-term survival (years)
A (radical nephrectomy + lymphadenectomy)	531 (51%)	55.5 ± 10	18	57 ± 6
B (radical nephrectomy + node biopsy)	199 (19%)	60.3 ± 1	6	50 ± 12
C (radical nephrectomy alone)	305 (29%)	66.5 ± 11	3	44 ± 9

Based on Schaufhauser et al. (1999).
* Number in parenthesis is the percentage of patients of the total in each cohort.

The mean follow-up for these groups of patients was 115 months ± 63 months. After disease stage matching, group A was found to have the least favourable tumour stage, but nevertheless long-term survival in this group was most favourable. Of lymph node-positive cases in group A, 27% were alive at 5 years. The authors concluded that approximately 4% of patients benefit from lymphadenectomy. This is a small number but the authors suggest that, for these lymph node-positive patients, there is a significant additional chance of survival.

Herrlinger et al. (1991) reported a prospective study of 511 patients being treated by extended dissection of retroperitoneal nodes with radical nephrectomy or radical nephrectomy, with 'facultative dissection' of nodes for staging purposes if the surgeon considered them macroscopically involved. The 5-year survival rate for these two groups was 66% versus 58% and 10-year survival rates of 56% versus 41% respectively. Patients with pT1–2 and pT3N0M0 disease were found to derive the greatest benefit from extended lymphadenectomy. Operative mortality was found to be lower (< 1%) following lymphadenectomy than for more conservative surgery. Herrlinger concluded that radical nephrectomy with curative intentions should include extended dissection of the lymph nodes. Unfortunately, no information is given as to how the two groups were selected or that they were comparable in age, follow-up and preoperative performance status. Most importantly, there is no confirmation of comparable disease stage between the two groups or that similar proportions of lymph node-positive patients were in both arms of the study.

Debate as to the benefit of lymphadenectomy will continue, but this is one area that has been investigated using a prospective randomised trial conducted by the European Organisation for Research and Treatment of Cancer (EORTC) – Phase III Protocol 30881. Preliminary results were published in 1999 (Blom et al. 1999) but no survival data are yet available. The trial has randomised 772 patients with resectable, non-metastatic RCC to complete lymph node dissection with radical nephrectomy or radical nephrectomy alone. Preliminary results show that the surgical complication rate between the two groups did not differ statistically significantly (25.7 and 22.2% respectively). Lymph node dissection does not therefore increase morbidity or mortality, but longer follow-up is required to assess its efficacy in terms of prolonged tumour-free survival and local recurrence.

The evidence for adrenalectomy as part of radical nephrectomy for renal carcinoma

As noted above, Robson (1969) popularised removal of the ipsilateral adrenal as part of radical nephrectomy. The removal of the adrenal appears logical in an attempt to remove all disease that may have extended locally from, for example, upper pole tumours. Furthermore, the shared venous drainage of the left adrenal and kidney raises the possibility of retrograde flow, allowing tumour implantation from the primary into the adrenal. Further justification for en bloc adrenalectomy could come from evidence of metastatic disease, to the ipsilateral adrenal, with predictable frequency.

The incidence of involvement of the ipsilateral adrenal varies from series to series and is different in post mortem (29%) and clinical reports. Shalev et al. (1995) summarised 1932 patients from various surgical series and noted an overall incidence of 4.1% with a range of 1.2–8.3%. Tsui et al. (2000b) recently reported on a single centre series of 511 patients treated over a 12-year period. All patients had ipsilateral adrenalectomy, 164 patients had 'localised' and 347 'advanced' disease. The overall incidence of adrenal involvement 29 of 511 (5.7%).

The incidence of adrenal involvement was related to the T category and increased from 0.6% for T1–2 to 7.8% for T3 and 40% for T4 primary tumours. The risk factors for adrenal involvement included higher T category, upper pole location of the primary tumour, the presence of multi-focal tumours and venous extension from the primary tumour. Preoperative CT had a negative predictive value of 99.4%, although the CT review was not masked in this study.

By contrast, Knobloch et al. (1999) reported that preoperative CT was not reliable in the detection of adrenal involvement. These authors found adrenal metastases in 19 of 589 (3.2%) patients having nephrectomy and ipsilateral adrenalectomy between 1985 and 1997. They also found that the incidence increased with increasing T category. For tumours ≤ pT2 the incidence was 0.9% and for tumours ≥ pT3 the incidence was 6.6%. There was no correlation of tumour site and adrenal involvement in their series. Different authors disagree on the correlation of primary tumour site and size, and the presence of adrenal metastases (Table 6.10).

Table 6.10 Incidence of adrenal metastases in surgical series

Author	No of patients	Incidence of adrenal tumour (%)	No. of lesions from T1/2 primary	Site of primary considered important	Size of primary considered important
Kletscher et al. (1996)	100	2	1/2	No	No
Shalev et al. (1995)	285	3.8	0/285	Yes	No
Sagalowsky et al. (1994)	695	4.3	4/327	No	No
Tsui et al. (2000b)	511	5.7	1/164	Yes	No

Comparative studies in the management of the ipsilateral adrenal

An Austrian retrospective, multicentre study of 225 patients having nephrectomy for unilateral renal tumours performed either with (109 patients) or without (116 patients) adrenalectomy has been reported. The two groups were matched for sex, age, laterality and nodal status, but were not randomised. The mean follow-up time was 78 months. Eight patients (8/109) had adrenal involvement. There was no significant survival difference for patients having T1–2 tumours. Overall, adrenalectomy was not considered to be of any benefit (Kozak et al. 1996). There are no meta-analyses and no randomised trials reporting nephrectomy with or without adrenalectomy.

In summary, for the patient with a normal ipsilateral adrenal on preoperative CT and a low stage tumour (T1 or T2), the risk of leaving disease, by not removing the adrenal, is very low. Any planned randomised study, whether or not designed to address the question of en bloc removal, should take into account the overall low incidence of adrenal involvement and the need for long follow-up.

Evidence for benefit of vena caval extraction

Renal cell carcinoma, in common with some other tumours, such as adrenal cortical carcinoma, has a predilection for growth along the venous drainage. Microscopic evidence of venous invasion or extension is common. In approximately 4–13% of patients, there may be extension out of the main renal vein and into the vena cava. The presence of this vena caval extension can represent a considerable challenge for the surgeon. Untreated, such disease may obstruct the vena cava, or in some patients segments of tumour or thrombus, on the surface of the tumour, may fragment and result in pulmonary emboli. Extension into the atrium may compromise cardiac function and may result in cardiac failure.

A variety of studies has investigated the impact of major venous extension on the prognosis. The presence of venous extension alone, or the cranial limit of the extension, does not necessarily diminish survival if complete surgical excision can be achieved. Invasion of the wall of the vena cava (Hatcher et al. 1991) or the presence of lymph nodes (Kuczyk et al. 1997) has a marked detrimental effect on survival. The presence of distant metastases in association with major venous extension also has a significant impact on survival (Swierzewski et al. 1994).

The evidence for a benefit from surgical intervention comes from descriptive studies of surgical series. Without intervention, most patients will die within a few months. There are no available randomised studies comparing intervention with no intervention. The ethics of such studies would be controversial, with the possible exception of patients having metastatic disease in association with vena caval extension.

The first report of long-term survival, after extraction of vena caval thrombus, appeared in 1956 (Skinner et al. 1972). Before this most reports were of death during or after the procedure.

Preoperative evaluation is of great importance because the presence of metastatic disease represents a contraindication to surgery in asymptomatic patients. Accurate assessment of the extent of the intraluminal tumour thrombus is fundamental because this determines the surgical approach, the position of the patient on the table and the need for cardiopulmonary bypass. There have been improvements in surgical technique and perioperative care and a major leap forward for patients with level IV extension came with the introduction of effective cardiopulmonary bypass with deep hypothermic arrest procedures. The classification of the level of extension is shown in Table 6.11.

Table 6.11 Classification of the level of venous extension

Level I	Thrombi (< 2 cm from renal venous ostium)
Level II	Thrombi (> 2 cm from venous ostium, below the hepatic veins)
Level III	Thrombi (tumour above the hepatic veins but below the cavoatrial junction)
Level IV	Thrombi (in the right atrium)

The approach to level III tumour thrombi is probably the most controversial, and a variety of surgical techniques to excise these tumours has been described.

The main issues in resection of level III tumours include the fact that clamping the vena cava in its intrapericardial portion can compromise venous return to the heart. Subsequent decreased cardiac output, haemodynamic instability and hypoperfusion of vital organs may occur unless the aorta is controlled as well. Cross-clamping the vena cava can also produce significant haemorrhage from venous collaterals which is often difficult to control. A trial of cross-clamping may be attempted to see how well the obstruction of the cava is tolerated.

Paradoxically, resection of a tumour that is obstructing the vena cava is usually better tolerated because chronic obstruction probably leads to the development of a collateral network, which is able to provide sufficient return of blood.

For tumours that extend to the right atrium, it is necessary to use cardiopulmonary bypass. Conventionally this involves median sternotomy and full exposure of the heart, although a minimal access approach with a small right subclavicular incision to access the right subclavian artery for arterial access, rather than the traditional aortic arch approach and a right parasternal incision to access the right atrium, has been described (Fitzgerald et al. 1998).

The outcome in terms of 5- and, where available, 10-year survival is summarised in Table 6.12.

Table 6.12 Survival after surgery for vena caval extension

Author	No. of patients	5-year survival rate (%)	10-year survival rate (%)
Skinner et al. (1989)	53		
All patients		29	NA
M1		0	0
Swierzewski et al. (1994)	100		
M0N0	72	64	57
M1	28	19.6	0
Hatcher et al. (1991)	44		
M0N0 42			
M1 13			

Conclusions and recommendations

The Oxford Centre for Evidence-based Medicine Levels of Evidence (May 2001) can be applied to the above observations as follows:

- Simple nephrectomy improves survival over conservative management (level 4).
- Simple nephrectomy has apparent poor 5-year survival rates for stage II disease (level 4).
- Radical nephrectomy may improve survival over simple nephrectomy in stage I and II disease (level 4).
- The full extent of any advantage of radical nephrectomy over simple nephrectomy remains controversial.

- Radical nephrectomy is a safe operation with excellent local control and survival rates in specialist centres (level 2c).
- Survival rates for localised and locally advanced disease appear to be improving over time (level 4).
- Lymphadenectomy does not increase morbidity or mortality (level 1b).
- Retrospective and non-randomised studies suggest that lymphadenectomy plus radical nephrectomy improves survival when compared with radical nephrectomy alone (level 3b).
- Survival results of a completed prospective randomised trial are not yet available.
- The benefit of adrenalectomy is very small for T1 and T2 tumours (level 3b).
- Long-term survival can be achieved for patients with extension to the vena cava.
- Complete surgical excision and the absence of lymph node or distant metastases are important components for such long-term survival (level 2c).

The introduction of new surgical techniques for localised disease should be considered an opportunity to improve the levels of evidence for surgical intervention.

References

Blom JHM, van Poppel H, Marechal JM et al. (1999) Radical nephrectomy with and without lymph node dissection: preliminary results of the EORTC randomised phase III protocol 30881. *European Urology* **36**: 570–575.

Corman JM, Penson DF, Hur K et al. (2000) Comparison of complications after radical and partial nephrectomy: results from the National Veterans Administration Surgical Quality Improvement Program. *British Journal of Urology International* **86**: 782–789.

Chute R, Soutter L, Kerr WS Jr (1949) The value of thoraco-abdominal incision in removal of kidney tumours. *New England Journal of Medicine* **241**: 951.

de Kernion JB (1980) Lymphadenectomy for renal cell carcinoma: therapeutic implications. *Urologic Clinics of North America* **7**: 697–703.

de Kernion JB, Ramming KP, Smith RB (1978) The natural history of metastatic renal cell carcinoma: a computer analysis. *Journal of Urology* **120**: 148–152.

Dinney CP, Awad SA, Gaewski JB et al. (1992) Analysis of imaging modalities, staging systems and prognostic indicators for renal cell carcinoma. *Urology* **39**: 122–129.

Fitzgerald JM, Tripathy U, Svenson LG et al. (1998) Radical nephrectomy with vena caval thrombectomy using a minimal access approach for cardiopulmonary bypass. *Journal of Urology* **159**: 1292–1293.

Flocks RH, Kadesky MC (1958) Malignant neoplasms of the kidney: an analysis of 353 patients followed for five years or more. *Journal of Urology* **79**: 196.

Giberti C, Oneto F, Martorana G, Rovida S, Carmignani G (1997) Radical nephrectomy for renal cell carcinoma: long term results and prognostic factors in a series of 328 cases. *European Urology* **31**: 40–48.

Giuliani L, Martorana G, Giberti C et al. (1983) Results of radical nephrectomy with extensive lymphadenectomy for renal cell carcinoma. *Journal of Urology* **130**: 664–668.

Golimbu M, Joshi P, Sperber M, Tessler A, Al-Askari S, Morales P (1986) Renal cell carcinoma: survival and prognostic factors. *Urology* **17**: 291–301.

Guinan PD, Vogelzang NJ, Fremgen A et al. (1995) Renal cell carcinoma: tumour size, stage and survival. *Journal of Urology* **153**: 901–903.

Hatcher PA, Anderson EE, Paulson DF et al. (1991) Surgical management and prognosis of renal cell carcinoma invading the vena cava. *Journal of Urology* **145**: 20–24.

Herrlinger A, Schrott KM, Schott G, Sigel A (1991) What are the benefits of extended dissection of the regional lymph nodes in the therapy of renal cell carcinoma? *Journal of Urology* **146**: 1224–1227

Hofmockel G, Tsatalpas P, Muller H (1995) Significance of conventional and new prognostic factors for locally confined renal cell carcinoma. *Cancer* **76**: 296.

Humphreys GA, Foot NC (1960) Survival of patients following nephrectomy for renal cell carcinoma and treatment of transitional cell tumours of the kidney. *Journal of Urology* **83**: 815–819

Kletscher BA, Qian J, Bostwick DG et al. (1996) Prospective analysis of the incidence of ipsilateral adrenal metastasis in localised renal cell carcinoma. *Journal of Urology* **155**: 1844–1846

Knobloch R, Seseke F, Riedmiller H et al. (1999) Radical nephrectomy for renal cell carcinoma: is adrenalectomy necessary? *European Urology* **36**: 303–308.

Kozak W, Holtl W, Pummer K, Maier U, Jeschke K, Bucher A (1996) Adrenalectomy – still a must in radical renal surgery? *British Journal of Urology* **77**(1): 27–31.

Kuczyk MA, Bokemeyer C, Kohn G et al. (1997) Prognostic relevance of intracaval neoplastic extension for patients with renal cell cancer. *British Journal of Urology* **80**: 18–24.

Ljungberg B, Alamdari FI, Holmberg G, Granfors T, Duchek M (1998) Radical nephrectomy is still preferable in the treatment of localized renal cell carcinoma. *European Urology* **33**: 79–85.

McNichols DW, Segura JW, de Weerd JH (1981) Renal cell carcinoma: long term survival and late recurrence. *Journal of Urology* **126**: 17–23.

Middleton RG, Presto AJ (1973) Radical thoracoabdominal nephrectomy for renal cell carcinoma. *Journal of Urology* **110**: 36.

Mintz ER, Gaul EA (1939) Kidney tumours: some causes of poor end results. *New York Journal of Medicine* **39**: 1405–1411.

Mortensen H (1948) Transthoracic nephrectomy. *Journal of Urology* **60**: 855.

Priestley JT (1939) Survival following the removal of malignant renal neoplasms. *Journal of the American Medical Association* **113**: 902–906.

Ramon J, Goldwasser B, Raviv G, Jonas P, Many M (1990) Long term results of simple and radical nephrectomy for renal cell carcinoma. *Cancer* **67**: 2506–2511.

Riches E, Griffiths JM, Thackray AC (1951) New growths of the kidney and ureter. *British Journal of Urology* **23**: 297–351.

Robson CJ, Churchill BM, Anderson W (1969) The results of radical nephrectomy for renal cell carcinoma. *Journal of Urology* **101**: 297–301.

Sagalowsky AI, Kadesky KT, Ewalt DM et al. (1994) Factors influencing adrenal metastasis in renal cell carcinoma. *Journal of Urology* **151**: 1181–1184.

Schaufhauser W, Ebert A, Brod J, Petsch S, Schrott K (1999) Lymph node involvement in renal cell carcinoma and survival chance by systematic lymphadenectomy. *Anticancer Research* **19**(2C): 1573–1578.

Shalev M, Cipolla B, Guille F et al. (1995) Is ipsilateral adrenalectomy a necessary component of radical nephrectomy? *Journal of Urology* **153**: 1415–1417.

Siatoh H (1982) Distant metastasis of renal adenocarcinoma in nephrectomized cases. *Journal of Urology* **127**: 1092–1095.

Siow WY, Yip SKH, Ng LG, Tan PH, Cheng Ws, Foo KT (2000) Renal cell carcinoma: incidental detection and pathological staging. *Journal of the Royal College of Surgeons of Edinburgh* **45**: 291–295.

Skinner DG, Colvin RB, Vermillion CD, Pfister RC, Leadbetter WF (1971) Diagnosis and management of renal cell carcinoma: a clinical and pathologic study of 309 cases. *Cancer* **28**: 1165–1177.

Skinner DG, Pfister R, Colvin RB et al. (1972a) Extension of renal cell carcinoma into the vena cava: the rationale for aggressive surgical management. *Journal of Urology* **107**: 711–716.

Skinner, DG, Vermillion CD, Colvin RB et al. (1972b) The surgical management of renal cell carcinoma. *Journal of Urology* **107**: 705–710.

Skinner D, Pritchett T, Lieskovsky G et al. (1989) Vena caval involvement by renal cell carcinoma. Surgical resection provides meaningful long-term survival. *Annals of Surgery* **210**: 387–394.

Swierzewski D, Swierzewski M, Libertino JK et al. (1994) Radical nephrectomy in patients with renal cell carcinoma with venous, vena caval and atrial extension. *American Journal of Surgery* **168**: 205–209.

TNM (1997) *Classification of Malignant Tumours*, 5th edn. Geneva: UICC (International Union Against Cancer).

Tsui K, Shvarts O, Smith R, Figlin R, de Kernion JB, Belldegrun A (2000a) Prognostic indicators for renal cell carcinoma: a multivariate analysis of 643 patients using the revised 1997 TNM staging criteria. *Journal of Urology* **163**: 1090–1095.

Tsui K, Shvarts O, Barbaric Z, Figlin R, de Kernion JB, Belldegrun A (2000b) Is adrenalectomy a necessary component of radical nephrectomy? UCLA experience with 511 radical nephrectomies. *Journal of Urology* **163**: 437–441.

Wood DP, Herr HW (1989) The evolving role of surgery in the management of renal cell carcinoma. *Seminars in Urology* **8**: 172–180.

Zisman A, Pantuck A, Belldegrun AS (2003) The role of retroperitoneal lymph node disection in a comprehensive approach to renal cell carcinoma. (In the press.)

Chapter 7

The evidence base of nephron-sparing surgery: surgical techniques and an evaluation of their clinical outcome

Michael Aitchison and Emma Bromwich

For the past 30 years radical nephrectomy has been the gold standard treatment for renal cell carcinoma (RCC) and provides the best hope for cure of organ-confined disease (Robson et al. 1969). To avoid renal dialysis in patients with tumours in a solitary kidney, the technique of partial nephrectomy or nephron-sparing surgery has been developed over the past 20 years. Nephron-sparing surgery (NSS) has become the recommended surgical option for patients with bilateral renal tumours (including patients with von Hippel–Lindau disease), tumours in a solitary kidney or a unilateral tumour with already compromised renal function.

The increasing availability and utilisation of modern non-invasive imaging techniques (ultrasonography, computed tomography [CT] and magnetic resonance imaging [MRI]) has resulted in increasing numbers of small, incidental, asymptomatic RCCs being detected. Several authors have advocated extending the indications for NSS to include such patients with small tumours and a normal contralateral kidney (Morgan and Zincke 1990; Steinbach et al. 1992; Licht et al. 1994; Butler et al. 1995). The increasing frequency of partial nephrectomy as a surgical treatment of patients with tumours ≤ 2.5 cm, identified in the Nation Cancer Database, suggests that this widening of the indication for NSS has gained widespread acceptance in the urological community (Marshall et al. 1997).

Nephron-sparing surgery as a cancer operation

Improved survival in patients treated with radical rather than simple nephrectomy has never been demonstrated in a randomised controlled clinical trial. NSS, however, by leaving *in situ* the affected kidney, does run the risk of local tumour recurrence. To qualify as a viable alternative to radical or simple nephrectomy, NSS must demonstrate a similar complication rate, local recurrence rate and cancer-specific survival.

Surgical complication rate

It is noteworthy that most authors have concentrated on survival and recurrence rates rather than surgical complications of this technically demanding and relatively rarely performed procedure. Two series, specifically addressing complications, both clearly identify a learning curve phenomenon, with a significant decrease in the complication rate with increasing experience with the technique (Campbell et al. 1994; Polaschik et al. 1995).

Urinary fistula formation is the most common complication (10–17%). Central tumour location, tumour size > 4 cm, ex vivo surgery and major reconstruction of the collecting system are all risk factors for this complication. Tumours < 4 cm have a lower risk of fistula formation (8.8% – Campbell et al. 1994). The majority of fistulae resolve spontaneously; the remainder can be dealt with by endoscopic means (stent or percutaneous drainage).

Renal failure can occur in up to a quarter of patients with a solitary functioning kidney who have NSS and risk factors for this complication are large tumours > 7 cm, multiple tumours, central location of the tumour and a long ischaemic time. Postoperative renal failure usually resolves and only 5% of patients require permanent dialysis (Campbell et al. 1994).

In patients with pre-existing renal impairment, postoperative renal failure is uncommon (2%), but with continued deterioration in renal function more patients may require subsequent permanent dialysis (Polaschik et al. 1995).

Postoperative haemorrhage and perinephric abscess are reported to occur in 6% and 7% of cases, but can be treated by embolisation and percutaneous drainage (Campbell et al. 1994).

Campbell and Novick's series of 259 patients, in 1994, represents the largest series and quotes a perioperative mortality rate of 1.5%, with 3.1% of complications requiring repeat open surgery. The complication rates in all series increase with the size of the tumour and the location (peripheral vs central)

No randomised study comparing complications of radical nephrectomy versus NSS exists. Single institution studies with matched patient groups suggest that the complication rates of the two procedures are similar at least in small (< 4 cm) tumours (Hafez et al. 1998).

Local recurrence rates

The local recurrence rate following NSS may be determined by two factors: first, an inadequate excision of the tumour may leave positive microscopic surgical margins or, second, there may be small foci of tumour elsewhere in the kidney, i.e. multifocal tumour. The first factor is related to the technique of NSS and can be avoided by excision rather than enucleation and histological confirmation of excision margin by frozen section. The second factor, multifocality of tumours, represents the major disadvantage of NSS.

The incidence of multifocality of renal tumours has been reported to be as high as 20% (Mukamel et al. 1988), but more detailed studies have shown that the incidence of multifocality is related to the size of the primary tumour, with an incidence of 7% in tumours < 8 cm (Cheng et al. 1991). A detailed prospective study with 3-mm step sectioning of radical nephrectomy specimens identified a 6% incidence of multifocal areas of tumour that had not been detected on preoperative imaging (Kletscher et al. 1995).

The local recurrence rates quoted in series with long-term follow-up of significant numbers of patients post-NSS range from 0% to 6% (Herr 1999; Lerner et al. 1996; Hafez et al. 1997). Tumours < 4 cm have recurrence rates of 4.6% (Lerner et al. 1996), and 0% recurrence rates are quoted for tumours < 2.5 cm (Herr 1999; Hafez et al. 1998).

The detailed follow-up of patients undergoing NSS because of the concern over local recurrence caused by multifocality has, paradoxically, highlighted the incidence of contralateral tumour recurrence in patients undergoing nephrectomy for unilateral renal cell cancer which ranges from 4% to 7% in patients followed for at least 10 years (Dehcit et al. 1998; Herr 1999). This has been used by proponents of NSS to support the argument for NSS for small tumours in patients with a normal contralateral kidney.

Survival after nephron-sparing surgery

A prospective, randomised controlled, clinical trial is required to determine scientifically whether NSS is comparable to radical nephrectomy in terms of survival. Such a trial was commenced in 1992 under the auspices of the European Organisation for Research and Treatment of Cancer (EORTC; study coordinator HV Poppel) and has now become an intergroup study. Patients with tumours < 5 cm are randomised to NSS and limited lymphadenectomy or radical nephrectomy and limited lymphadenectomy. The low incidence of recurrence and the expected high 5- to 10-year survival rates require a large number of patients to be randomised (1300) to achieve adequate statistical power. This factor and the advent of laparoscopic nephrectomy have led to a lengthy recruitment period and an uncertain closure date.

In the absence of randomised control data, the literature provides level III-type evidence from comparative single institution studies: a 97% 10-year cancer specific survival rate in 67 patients treated with NSS for tumours < 7 cm has been reported (Herr 1999), and a 94.5% 10-year cancer-specific survival rate in 43 patients with tumours < 4 cm. Comparing 185 NSS-treated patients with 209 matched patients treated with radical nephrectomy showed no difference in cancer-specific survival in patients with tumours < 4 cm (Lerner et al. 1996).

Nephron-sparing surgery in von Hippel–Lindau disease

Of patients with von Hippel–Lindau disease, 45% develop RCC and these lesions are frequently multifocal and bilateral (Maher et al. 1990). NSS has been shown to provide effective initial treatment in such patients with 5-year and 10-year cancer-specific survival rates of 100% and 81%. Local recurrence and the development of new tumours are inevitable and careful follow-up, repeat surgery and eventually radical nephrectomy may be required (Steinback et al. 1995).

Technique of nephron-sparing surgery

Various operative techniques have been described but the series of over 500 patients from the Cleveland Clinic of Dr Andrew Novick represents the largest single series with detailed description of operative technique and surgical complications.

Detailed preoperative radiological investigation using CT with three-dimensional reconstruction, selective renal angiography or magnetic resonance angiography to identify the extra- and intrarenal vascular anatomy can be performed. These intensive investigations may not be for small peripheral tumours, but aid planning surgery in large central tumours in a solitary kidney.

An extraperitoneal flank incision through or between the eleventh and twelfth ribs provides good access, and allows mobilisation of the kidney and removal of the perinephric fat, except over the area of the tumour, for inspection of the renal surface to exclude any peripheral multifocal tumour deposits.

Mobilisation of the renal vessels allows for both arterial and venous occlusion if necessary. Small peripheral tumours may be excised without any vessel occlusion, but larger or centrally placed tumours require arterial and venous occlusion to allow a bloodless field for adequate excision and repair of the renal defect. Mannitol is given before arterial occlusion and surface cooling of the kidney with ice for 10–15 minutes results in a core renal temperature of 15–20°C to allow *in situ* renal preservation (Licht et al. 1994; Campbell and Novick 1995).

Intraoperative ultrasonography is useful to localise the intrarenal extent of tumours (Campbell et al. 1996). Frozen section analysis of the resection margin should be used to confirm surgical clearance (Campbell et al. 1996).

Control of the vascular pedicle allows for precise closure of the collecting system and haemostasis by suture ligation of cut vessels. The renal defect can be closed or covered with surrounding tissue or artificial haemostatic material. Some authors use methylene blue injection of the collecting system to confirm closure of the collecting system and routine ureteric stenting (Polaschik et al. 1995), but this is not felt to be necessary by others (Campbell et al. 1996).

Ex vivo or bench surgery with autotransplantation has been described (Morgan and Zincke 1990; Campbell et al. 1994), for large tumours in solitary kidneys. This technique has a higher complication and recurrence rate and, with increasing surgical experience of *in situ* partial nephrectomy, it appears to have been largely abandoned.

Laparoscopic partial nephrectomy

With increasing numbers of radical nephrectomies being performed for renal malignancy, specialised centres have turned to partial laparoscopic nephrectomy as an alternative to the open technique. In a review of the European experience, Rassweiller et al. (2000) describe the experience in 53 cases from four centres with an average tumour size of 2.3 cm (range 1.1–5 cm). The technical complexity of the procedure led to an 8% open conversion rate and two complete nephrectomies. The technical problems related to haemorrhage and persistent urinary leak. This high incidence of complications should decrease with experience and improvements in technique, but at present this advanced laparoscopic technique should be restricted to centres with considerable experience in laparoscopy. Median follow-up of 24 months is too short to provide reassurance that this is an adequate tumour operation, and further experience and longer follow-up are required to ascertain whether tumour cell spillage might result in high local recurrence rates. The mean time to recurrence in open partial nephrectomy is 42 months (Hafez et al. 1999).

Application of new technologies to partial nephrectomy technique

Ablation of tumours, particularly small peripheral tumours, has been attempted using a variety of technologies such as high-intensity focused ultrasonography in experimental models and cryotherapy (Chan et al. 1999; Patel et al. 1999; Chen et al. 2000).

The problem with any technique that destroys a tumour *in situ* is the adequacy of tumour destruction and the interpretation of follow-up scans. The largest published series of laparoscopic cryoablation consists of 35 patients with small peripheral tumours (mean diameter 2–3 cm, range 1–3 cm); follow-up with MRI and CT biopsy of the cryolesions reveals no local recurrence at a mean follow-up of 11.2 months (Chen et al. 2000).

All these novel treatments may have advantages over open partial nephrectomy, but careful patient selection and lengthy follow-up with a clinical trial situation are required to demonstrate their efficacy and safety.

Conclusion

The technique of NSS has evolved and improved over the last 25 years and it is now established as the treatment of choice in patients with tumours in a solitary kidney. The surgical results, local recurrence rates and cancer -specific survival for tumours > 4 cm in patients with a normal contralateral kidney are comparable to that for radical nephrectomy, although this has not been tested in a randomised controlled clinical trial. New surgical techniques combined with new technologies may provide alternatives to open partial nephrectomy, but careful evaluation and long follow-up are required.

References

Butler B, Novick AC, Miller D, Campbell Sc, Licht MR (1995) Management of small unilateral renal cell carcinomas. Radical versus nephron sparing surgery. *Urology* **45**: 34–40.
Campbell SC, Novick AC (1995) Surgical technique and morbidity of elective partial nephrectomy. *Seminars in Urologic Oncology* **13**: 281.

Campbell SC, Novick AC, Streem SB, Klein E, Licht M (1994) Complications of nephron sparing surgery for renal tumours. *Journal of Urology* **151**: 1177–1180.

Campbell SC, Fichtner J, Novick AC et al. (1996) Intraoperative evaluation of renal cell carcinoma. A prospective study of the role of ultrasonography and histopathological frozen sections. *Journal of Urology* **155**: 1191–1195.

Chan D, Pant B, Pacheco R et al. (1999) Power requirements for renal ablation using high intensity focussed ultrasound in a rabbit model (abstract). *Journal of Endourology* 13: A13.

Chen RN, Novick AC, Gill IS (2000) Laparoscopic cryoablation of renal masses. *Urologic Clinics of North America* **27**: 813–820.

Cheng WS, Farrow GM, Zincke H (1991) The incidence of multicentricity in renal cell carcinoma. *Journal of Urology* **146**: 1221.

Dehcit CB, Blute ML, Zincke H (1998) Nephron sparing surgery for unilateral renal cell carcinoma: which pathological variables contribute to contralateral tumour recurrence. *Journal of Urology* **159**: 648.

Hafez KS, Novick AC, Butler BP (1998) Management of small solitary unilateral renal cell carcinomas: impact of central versus peripheral tumour locations. *Journal of Urology* **159**: 1156–1160.

Hafez KS, Fergany AF, Novick AC (1999) Nephron sparing surgery for localised renal cell carcinoma: impact of recurrence on patient survival, tumour recurrence and TNM staging. *Journal of Urology* **162**: 1930–1933.

Herr HW (1999) Partial nephrectomy for unilateral renal cell carcinoma and a normal unilateral renal cell carcinoma and a normal contralateral kidneys: 10 year follow up. *Journal of Urology* **161**: 33–35.

Kletscher BA, Quian J, Bostwick DG, Andrews PE, Zincke H (1995) Prospective analysis of multifocality in renal cell carcinoma: influence of histological pattern, grade, number, size, volume and deoxyribonucleic acid ploidy. *Journal of Urology* **153**: 904.

Lerner SC, Hawkins CA, Blute ML et al. (1996) Disease outcome in patients with low stage renal cell carcinoma treated with nephron sparing or radical surgery. *Journal of Urology* **155**: 1858.

Licht MR, Novick AC, Goornastic M (1994) Nephron sparing surgery in incidental versus suspected renal cell carcinoma. *Journal of Urology* **152**: 39–42.

Maher ER, Yates JR, Harries R et al. (1990) Clinical features and natural history of von Hippel–Lindau disease. *Quarterly Journal of Medicine* **238**: 1151.

Marshall FF, Stewart AK, Menck HR (1997) The Nation Cancer Data Base: Report on kidney carcinoma. *Cancer* **80**: 2167–2174.

Morgan WR, Zincke H (1990) Progression and survival after renal conserving surgery for renal cell carcinoma: Experience in 104 patients and extended follow up. *Journal of Urology* **144**: 852–857.

Mukamel E, Konicherty M, Engelstein D, Servadio C (1998) Incidental small renal tumours accompanying clinically overt renal cell carcinoma. *Journal of Urology* **140**: 22.

Patel VR, Leveillee RJ, Heran A et al. (1999) 'Wet' radiofrequency ablation of the rabbit kidney using the liquid electrode: Acute and chronic observations (abstract). *Journal of Endourology* **13**: A14.

Polaschik TJ, Pound CR, Meng MV, Porter AW, Marshall FF (1995) Partial nephrectomy: Techniques, complications and pathological findings. *Journal of Urology* **154**: 1312–1318.

Rassweiler JJ, Abbou C, Janetschek G, Jeschte K (2000) Laparoscopic partial nephrectomy. *Urologic Clinics of North America* **27**: 721–736.

Robson CJ, Churchill BM, Anderson W (1969) The results of radical nephrectomy for renal cell carcinoma. *Journal of Urology* **101**: 297–303.

Steinbach F, Stockle M, Miller JW et al. (1992) Conservative surgery of renal cell tumours in 140 patients: 21 years of experience. *Journal of Urology* **148**: 24–29.

Chapter 8

The evidence base for laparoscopic approaches to renal cancer surgery: technical aspects and an evaluation of clinical outcome

Gareth E Jones and David A Tolley

Since the introduction of laparoscopic nephrectomy to the urologists' armamentarium by Clayman et al. (1990), numerous series have described this technique and its variations for both benign and malignant renal conditions. The German Urologic Association (Rassweiller et al. 1998a) described their experience of 482 procedures performed in 14 centres, with 444 of these for benign disease. Operative time ranged from 81.9 to 277.6 min and was dependent on surgeon's experience and the pathology of the resected organ. No significant variation in average operative time was noted. The complication rate was 6% and conversion to open surgery occurred in 10.3%. Secondary procedures were required in 3.4% and in six cases this was for bleeding. As yet, no randomised controlled data are available comparing laparoscopic and open nephrectomy; however, a number of comparative studies have been published. Rassweiller et al. (1998b) compared their experience with laparoscopy (both trans- and retroperitoneal routes) and open nephrectomy. Operative duration for both laparoscopic routes was roughly double that for open; postoperative analgesic requirements (2 vs 4 mg morphine) and convalescence (24 vs 40 days) were significantly lower in the laparoscopic groups and postoperative stay fell from 10 to 7 days. Fornera et al. (2001) describe equivalent operative time (90 min average) with decreased complications for the laparoscopic route (20% vs 25%), shorter hospital stay (4 vs 10 days) and shorter convalescence (24 vs 36 days). Conversion rates are reported as 6.1%. Our own experience of 200 laparoscopic nephrectomies is of a 19% complication rate (17% minor) and a conversion rate of 6.5%. With increasing experience, our operative duration fell from 204 to 108 min (first 50 vs second 50). Three major complications occurred during the first 100 cases, with only one in the second 100; no significant fall in minor complication rates was noted.

These facts provide evidence that laparoscopic renal surgery for benign renal disease is safe and superior to scalpel surgery, especially when postoperative factors such as pain, hospital stay and convalescence are taken into account. The work of Fornera et al. (2001) also indicates that with greater experience the principal problem with laparoscopic nephrectomy – operative time – becomes comparable with scalpel surgery. Table 8.1 summarises the advantages and disadvantages of laparoscopic nephrectomy. To extend the role of laparoscopy into malignant renal disease we must prove:

(1) equivalent or better surgical outcome
(2) equivalent oncological outcome.

Table 8.1 Advantages and disadvantages of laparoscopic renal surgery

Advantages	Disadvantages
Decreased blood loss	Technically demanding surgery
Lower postoperative analgesic requirement	Technology dependent
Shorter hospital stay	Steep learning curve for surgeon
Rapid return to normal activity	Long operative time
	High cost (disposable equipment)

Laparoscopic radical nephrectomy: technique

Radical nephrectomy mandates the removal of the kidney within Gerota's fascia along with the ipsilateral adrenal gland (Robson 1963). Laparoscopic extirpation has been described using the transperitoneal and retroperitoneal routes, along with the use of so-called hand-assisted techniques. Most series report transperitoneal surgery, stating ease of access, familiarity of anatomical landmarks and greater working space as technical benefits. The patient is placed in the flank position; the first 12-mm port is sited lateral to the rectus muscles at the level of the umbilicus using the Hassan technique, and then two further ports are sited in the anterior axillary line with transillumination to help avoid any significant vessels. A fourth port can be utilised in the mid-axillary line to facilitate retraction of intra-abdominal structures. The colon is reflected medially and the hilar vessels identified as in open nephrectomy. When adequately visualised, the hilar vessels are controlled (Endoclips for the renal artery and the Endo-GIA for the renal vein) and the kidney mobilised. The ureter is divided between Endoclips. Retroperitoneal laparoscopy requires the creation of a working cavity. In the flank position an initial incision anterior to the tip of the twelfth rib is deepened to allow insertion of a balloon dilator deep to the transversalis fascia (either home made with a Foley catheter and size 8 glove finger or purpose built); this is then inflated with 800 ml of saline for 5 min to create the working cavity.

Further ports are then sited as previously. Disadvantages of this technique are that landmarks are less obvious, the creation of a working cavity is time-consuming and inadvertent peritoneal injury will convert the technique to transperitoneal. Rassweiller et al. (1998b) and McDougall et al. (1996) reported slight benefits over transperitoneal laparoscopy, but less so than open surgery. Hand-assisted laparoscopy (HAL) combines the transperitoneal approach with the insertion of a larger port, to allow insertion of the surgeon's hand while the pneumoperitoneum is maintained.

This allows the surgeon the benefits of better vision (laparoscopy) and tactile feedback (open), and is best suited to procedures where an incision will be used to deliver the specimen. Wolf and Gill's (2001) editorial discusses their views on the role of HAL in urology. Batler et al. (2001) report six cases of HAL radical nephrectomy performed by residents with no laparoscopic experience; all were completed with an average operative time of 215 min and only one significant complication. The relative merits of each technique are summarised in Table 8.2.

Table 8.2 Comparison of laparoscopic routes

	Advantages	Disadvantages
Transperitoneal	Excellent view	Longer postoperative ileus
	Large working cavity	Adhesions may prove problematic
	Easily identifiable landmarks	Possible bowel/solid organ injury
		Peritoneal seeding of tumour possible
Retroperitoneal	Shorter ileus	Small working cavity
	Less analgesic use	Steeper learning curve
	Shorter hospital stay	Landmarks less apparent
		Peritoneal tearing can complicate the issue
Hand assisted (HA)	Excellent view	Port technology not yet perfect
	Direct tactile feedback during dissection	Large incision for HA laparoscopic port
	Relatively easy to learn	
	Intact specimen retrieval	

In our institution, after complete mobilisation of the specimen, we utilise the endocatch bag and extend the most convenient port site to extract the specimen intact. Other centres utilise lower midline, Pfannenstiel incisions or delivery via the vagina for small specimens has also been described. Savage and Gill (2001) observed no significant difference in postoperative factors utilising a muscle-splitting incision.

Barrett et al. (1998) and Landman et al. (2000) assess the effect of specimen morcellation. Pathological assessment of histological type, grade and stage were identical; however, exact tumour sizing was impossible after morcellation. Landman et al. (2000) also assessed the integrity of the laparoscopic retrieval bag after morcellation, and found no defects after morcellation of fresh tissue, although one sack of nine failed during morcellation of formalin-fixed tissue. This would tend to be reinforced by the lack of a single port site recurrence in the series of Barrett et al. (1998).

Clinical outcome of laparoscopic radical nephrectomy

When moving from laparoscopy for benign disease to radical surgery for cancer, concerns over adequacy of tumour excision (as reflected by local recurrence) and inadvertent tumour implantation must be addressed. The nephrectomy specimen from laparoscopic surgery includes the ipsilateral adrenal gland, perirenal fat and hilar nodes, and is comparable with that obtained from open radical nephrectomy; node dissection is also possible. Port site recurrence has been reported in two cases after tumour nephrectomy and in both these cases the specimen was morcellated before extraction and, in one ascites, was noted intraoperatively. Kavoussi et al. (1993) reported their initial experience of eight laparoscopic tumour nephrectomies with follow-up for 14 months and, to date, the longest available mean follow-up is 35.6 months. Since this time, more than 30 further reports have been published encompassing some 900 patients, with seven series reporting more than 50 patients, two series reporting 100 patients and one multicentre study. Overall a mean operative time of 176 min (range 125–308) has been noted with a complication rate of 3–35% (major 3–19%, minor 8–35%) and a conversion rate of 0–10%. Blood loss ranged from 128 to 320 ml. Hospital stay ranges from 1.6 to 10 days, although most recent series have an inpatient stay of fewer than 4 days. The time taken to return to normal activity in laparoscopic groups has been consistently reported in the range 21–25 days – roughly half that of the open surgical cohort.

Subgroup analysis of the Edinburgh series revealed 20 radical nephrectomies with an average operative time of 143 min and hospital stay averaging 5.5 days. Eight patients experienced minor complications and one patient, subsequently diagnosed as suffering from Zollinger–Ellison syndrome, perforated his duodenum postoperatively. One case required conversion as a result of adhesions. Mean tumour size in our series was 5.2 cm and histology revealed renal cell cancer in 19. To date we have noted no evidence of disease recurrence or progression.

Cadeddu et al. (1998) reported the experience from 1991 to 1997 of five centres worldwide: 157 patients with clinically localised renal cell cancer were identified, 64% of these had been followed up for a minimum of 1 year and 32% for 2 years, giving a mean duration of follow-up of 19.2 months. No cancer-specific deaths have occurred in this series; however, four patients have developed metastatic disease and one patient local recurrence. The authors quote a 91% actuarial 5-year survival rate. Gill et al. (2001) and Ono et al. (2001) both report large comparative series with 100/103 laparoscopic and 40/46 open radical procedures respectively. Gill describes his personal experience with retroperitoneal surgery of renal tumours with a mean size of 5.1 cm and a mean surgical time of 2.8 hours. Similar to our experience in benign disease, the surgical time fell in the second half of the series and was related to tumour size. The series from Nagoya describes tumours < 5 cm and show a mix of trans- and retroperitoneal techniques. Surgical times are longer at a mean of 4.7 hours; however, it is unclear whether this series includes multiple or trainee laparoscopists. Conversion rates are quoted at 2% and 3.8%, with similar blood loss (212 vs 254 ml). Interestingly, the majority of complications (14%) in Gill's series are reported as minor (11%); Ono's series describe a 13% complication rate with 6% requiring laparotomy (they do, however, count conversion as a complication). Follow-up in Gill's series is a mean of 16.1 months and in this time no local recurrences are noted and two patients developed metastatic disease. Three patients developed metastatic disease and one local recurrence in Ono's series, giving a 5-year disease-free survival rate of 95.1% (89.7% in the open group). The findings of all series reporting more than 50 patients are summarised in Tables 8.3 and 8.4.

Table 8.3 Laparoscopic radical nephrectomy series (surgical data)

Reference	n	Mean operative time (min)	Complications (%)	Conversion rate (%)	Mean blood loss (ml)
Nakada et al. (2001)	57	168	14	2	212
Ono et al. (2001)	103	282	13	3	254
Pavlovich et al. (2002)	61	330	37.7	1.6	172
Rasweiller et al. (1998a)	67	256	15	1.5	280
Rasweiller et al. (1998b)	73	142	12	Not stated	170
Rasweiller et al. (2000)	50	139	4	6	149

Table 8.4 Laparoscopic radical nephrectomy series (tumour/follow-up data)

Reference	Mean follow-up (months)	Outcome measures
Nakada et al. (2001)	16. 1	97% disease free 2 patients with metastases
Ono et al. (2001)	29	95% actuarial 5-year disease free
Pavlovich et al. (2002)	25	3% recurrent/metastatic disease
Rasweiller et al. (1998a)	35.6	95% disease free at 5 years 86% actuarial survival at 5 years
Rasweiller et al. (1998b)	13.3	No recurrent disease
Rasweiller et al. (2000)	Unclear	96% survival at 23 months

Nakada et al. (2001) reported their experience of HAL radical nephrectomy in a group of 18 patients, for tumours with a mean tumour diameter of 4.5 cm. A mean operative time of 220 min was noted. In this series, no formal conversions or re-explorations were required and, to date, no recurrent disease has been found. Although their operative time was roughly double that for open surgery, hospital stay (3.9 vs 5.1 days) and time to return to normal activity (15.8 vs 23.5 days) were significantly shorter.

Laparoscopic partial nephrectomy

With the increasing use of abdominal ultrasonography, a trend to early or incidental diagnosis of renal cell cancer has been noted. The work of Novack established partial nephrectomy as a reasonable alternative to radical nephrectomy for small renal tumours especially in the presence of compromised renal function, bilateral disease and in the solitary renal unit. Similar to open radical nephrectomy, a large loin incision and complete renal mobilisation are required. In an attempt to decrease the morbidity of a loin incision, laparoscopic partial nephrectomy has been investigated. Experience is relatively small, with only around 90 cases performed worldwide. Selective vascular clamping and renal cooling are inherent to open partial nephrectomy and, as yet, no reliable method has been developed in laparoscopy. Numerous energy sources have been utilised to combat the bleeding encountered when a normally perfused kidney is incised, including the harmonic scalpel, bipolar electrocautery, neodymium–YAG (yttrium–aluminium–garnet) laser and argon beam coagulator. To date, the largest review is reported by Rassweiller et al. (2000) with 53 patients using both retroperitoneal and transperitoneal renal mobilisation. Operative time averaged 191 min (range 90–320) with a mean blood loss of 725 ml (range 20–1500). The conversion rate was 8% with two patients converted for haemostasis and two as a result of inadequate tumour localisation. Two patients required secondary nephrectomy (one for bleeding) and, in total, six patients required secondary laparotomy. Postoperative complications occurred in 12%, most being urinary leakage/urinoma (10%). Histology revealed renal cell cancer in 69% of cases and, for these patients, the 3-year disease-free rate is stated at 100%.

Laparoscopically assisted ablative procedures

With the recent advances in laparoscopic technique and miniaturisation of ultrasound technology, intraoperative ultrasonography has become feasible. The difficulties inherent to the technique of laparoscopic partial nephrectomy sparked interest in alternative ablative techniques and, to date, radiofrequency energy and cryoablation have been applied to small renal masses in small, essentially experimental studies. Radiofrequency energy is applied percutaneously and Pavlovich et al. (2002) showed a small decrease in the size of renal masses, with a mean diameter of 2.4 mm pre-treatment at 2 months. Of the tumours, 79% showed non-enhancement on contrast computed tomography (CT) at this time. The authors state that this remains very much an experimental technique.

Chen et al. (2000) summarised the Cleveland Clinic technique and experience of laparoscopic cryoablation for small renal masses. They report the results in 35 patients with tumours 1–3 cm, who had an indication for nephron-sparing intervention or who had co-morbidity precluding radical surgery. Their operative time averaged 174 min and a mean blood loss of 85 ml was noted. A peroperative biopsy showed renal cancer in 68% of cases; 68% were discharged in less than 23 hours and two surgical complications were noted (liver laceration and retroperitoneal haematoma). Seventeen patients have been followed up for one year and all have had subsequent negative biopsies.

Evidence analysis of references

To date, the evidence for laparoscopic radical nephrectomy is based on relatively small numbers in centres with special interests (Table 8.5). The hope of recruiting patients to a randomised controlled trial is minimal in the age of the internet, given the publicity surrounding laparoscopy for benign disease. The data presented in all the laparoscopic series are relatively immature compared with those for open surgery, but do appear to be comparable if not superior.

Table 8.5 Level of evidence analysis (references)

Level of evidence (AHCPR 1992)	Reference
1a Meta-analysis of randomised trial (RT)	–
1b Analysis of RT	–
2a Non-randomised controlled study	–
2b 'Quasi-experimental' study	All the references
3 Case reports	Robson (1963); Clayman et al. (1991); Lalak et al. (2000)
4 'Authoritative' opinion	Dunn et al. (2000); Wolf and Gill (2001)

Conclusions

The data presented above confirm that laparoscopic approaches to renal cancer surgery are equivalent to open surgery as regards oncological control, and are associated with shorter hospital stay, less blood loss and a more rapid return to normal activity. Surgical time is initially significantly longer in the laparoscopic groups, but with increasing experience significant reductions do occur.

The lack of a randomised trial of laparoscopic versus open tumour nephrectomy, and the limited number of centres with sufficient experience, urge caution in the rapid general implementation of this technique. If a fully trained laparoscopic urologist is available, we would recommend this technique for all T1 tumours and T2 tumours < 10 cm in maximal diameter. The choice of laparoscopic approach should be based on the surgeon's preference and experience. We would recommend intact organ retrieval to allow accurate pathological staging. HAL techniques may assist the occasional or trainee laparoscopic surgeon; however, with increasing subspecialisation within urology, the trained laparoscopist and appropriate cross-subspeciality referral and training will remove the need for this halfway house. Laparoscopic partial nephrectomy and laparoscopically assisted tissue ablative procedures remain investigational at the beginning of 2002.

References

Barrett PH, Fentie DD, Taranger LA et al. (1998) Laparoscopic radical nephrectomy with morcellation for renal cell carcinoma: the Saskatoon experience. *Urology* 52: 23–82.

Batler RA, Schoor RA, Gonzalez CM et al. (2001) Hand-assisted laparoscopic radical nephrectomy: the experience of the inexperienced. *Journal of Endourology* 215: 513.

Cadeddu JA, Ono Y, Clayman RV et al. (1998) Laparoscopic nephrectomy for renal cell cancer: evaluation of efficacy and safety: a multicenter experience. *Urology* 52(5): 773–777.

Chan DY, Cadeddu JA, Jarrett TW et al. (2001) 100 laparoscopic radical nephrectomy: cancer control for renal cell carcinoma. *Journal of Urology* 166: 2095–2099.

Chen RN, Novick AC, Gill IS et al. (2000) Laparoscopic cryoablation of renal masses. *Urologic Clinics of North America* 27(4): 813–820.

Clayman RV, Kavoussi LR, Soper NJ et al. (1991) Laparoscopic nephrectomy: initial case report. *Journal of Urology* 146: 278.

Dunn MD, McDougall EM, Clayman RV et al. (2000) Laparoscopic radical nephrectomy. *Journal of Endourology* 14: 849–855.

Fornara P, Doehn C, Friedrich HJ et al. (2001) Non randomised comparison of open flank versus laparoscopic nephrectomy in 249 patients with benign renal disease. *European Urology* 40: 24–31.

Gill IS, Meraney AM, Schweizer DK et al. (2001) Laparoscopic radical nephrectomy in 100 patients. *Cancer* 92: 1843–1855.

Janetschek G, Jeschke K, Peschel R et al. (2000) Laparoscopic surgery for stage T1 renal cell carcinoma: radical nephrectomy and wedge resection. *European Urology* 38: 131–138.

Kavoussi LR, Kerbl K, Capelouto CC et al. (1993) Laparoscopic nephrectomy for renal neoplasms. *Urology* 42: 603–609.

Keeley FX, Tolley DA (1998) A review of our first 100 cases of laparoscopic nephrectomy: defining risk factors for complications. *British Journal of Urology* 82: 615–618.

Lalak N, Esposito M, Keeley FX et al. (2000) Complications of the first 200 cases of laparoscopic nephrectomy. *British Journal of Urology International* 88(suppl 1): 3.

Landman J, Lento P, Hassen W et al. (2000) Feasibility of pathological evaluation of morcellated kidneys after radical nephrectomy *Journal of Urology* 164: 2086–2089.

McDougall EM, Clayman RV et al. (1996) Laparoscopic nephrectomy for benign disease: comparison of the transperitoneal and retroperitoneal approaches. *Journal of Endourology* 10: 45–49.

Nakada SY, Fadden P, Jarrard DF et al. (2001) Hand assisted laparoscopic radical nephrectomy: comparison to open radical nephrectomy. *Urology* 58: 517–520.

Ono Y, Kinukawa T, Hattori R et al. (2001) The long-term outcome of laparoscopic radical nephrectomy for small renal cell carcinoma. *Journal of Urology* 165(6 Pt 1): 1867–1870.

Pavlovich CP, Walther MM, Choyke PL et al. (2002) Percutaneous radiofrequency ablation of small renal tumours: Initial results. *Journal of Urology* 167: 10–15.

Rassweiler J, Fornara P, Weber M et al. (1998a) Laparoscopic Nephrectomy: The experience of the laparoscopy working group of the German Urologic association. *Journal of Urology* 160(1): 18–21.

Rassweiler J, Frede T, Henkel TO et al. (1998b): Nephrectomy: A comparative study between the transperitoneal and retroperitoneal laparoscopic versus the open approach. *European Urology* 33: 489–496.

Rassweiler JJ, Abbou C, Janetschek G et al. (2000) Laparoscopic partial nephrectomy: The European experience. *Urologic Clinics of North America* **27**(4): 721–736.

Robson CJ (1963) Radical nephrectomy for renal cell cancer. *Journal of Urology* **89**: 37.

Savage SJ, Gill IS (2001) Intact specimen extraction during renal laparoscopy: muscle splitting versus muscle cutting incision. *Journal of Endourology* 15: 165–169.

Wolf JS Jr, Gill IS (2001) Editorial comment. *Urology* **58**: 310–317.

PART 4

Medical intervention

Chapter 9

Cytokine treatment in advanced renal cell carcinoma

Viviane Hess and Martin E Gore

In the UK, 5900 people are diagnosed with renal cell carcinoma (RCC) every year (Cancer Research Campaign 1999). Patients with localised disease can be cured by surgery; however, 20–30% of the patients who undergo radical nephrectomy for localised disease eventually relapse and die of their disease (3100 deaths from RCC per year – CRC 1999). One-third of newly diagnosed patients present with metastatic disease. The natural history of metastatic RCC can vary considerably from spontaneous remission (rare) to rapidly progressive disease; however, overall the prognosis is poor for these patients with a 5-year survival rate of less than 10% (Webb and Gore 2000).

RCC has always been regarded as a chemoresistant tumour. Phase II trials have shown some activity for 5-fluorouracil and vinblastine but only modestly so. Currently, there is no routine role for chemotherapy in the treatment of RCC, although relatively recent data suggest that some of the newer agents such as capecitabine (Wenzel et al. 2001) and gemcitabine (Casali et al. 2001) may produce responses.

Hormone treatment has also shown only minor objective anti-tumour activity in clinical trials. However, it can be of value as palliative treatment (e.g. as an appetite stimulant) and medroxyprogesterone acetate is frequently used for this purpose.

The variable natural history of metastatic renal cell cancer and the occasional spontaneous tumour regressions that occur suggests an important role for the immune system in controlling tumour growth and metastasis. Cytokines, such as the immunomodulatory proteins, interferons and interleukins, have therefore been used in the treatment of RCC. Immunotherapy is the only treatment modality that has been shown in randomised controlled trials to change the natural history of this disease and to provide survival benefit.

Interferons

Interferons (IFNs) are proteins secreted by various cells as a response to viral infection. There are three major classes of interferons: IFNα, -β and -γ.

IFNα and IFNβ are antiviral, being produced by infected cells and preventing the spread of infection to non-infected cells. Double-stranded RNA, which is not found in mammalian cells but in some viruses, is a potent inducer of IFN synthesis. IFNα and IFNβ bind to a common cellular receptor and activate a type of lymphocyte known as the natural killer (NK) cell. IFNγ is quite distinct. It is mainly produced by T cells as a response to specific antigen recognition and strongly activates macrophages.

The majority of clinical cancer research has centred on IFNα and to a lesser extent on IFNβ and IFNγ. All IFNs have a wide range of biological activity, including immunomodulation and antiviral, antiproliferative and anti-angiogenic effects. The precise mechanisms of their anti-tumour activity are only partly understood.

INFα is the only known treatment of advanced RCC that has demonstrated a survival benefit in randomised trials. However, the selection of those patients most likely to benefit from this and the optimum dose and duration of therapy still need to be investigated.

Interferon-β and interferon-γ

Interferon-β is not routinely used in cancer treatment. It was largely abandoned as a treatment for RCC, because Horoszewisz and Murphy (1989) showed in a cumulative analysis of phase II trials that INFα had a higher overall response rate (15% compared with 10% for INFβ). Similarly, IFNγ has shown to have no additional effect over placebo in a randomised controlled trial (Gleave et al. 1998).

Interferon-α

In the above-mentioned cumulative analysis (Horoszewicz and Murphy 1989), INFα as single agent therapy showed an overall response rate of 15% in a total of 1112 patients out of 33 trials. However, only 2% of patients obtained a complete response.

In the past, dosages of interferon varied considerably between different studies, although most trials used relatively high doses of INFα, i.e. > 10 MU/day. There is a suggestion from the early trials of a dose–response effect in that patients given < 3 MU/day of IFNα had an overall response of 12% and for those given 3–10 MU/day the overall response was 19%. The overall response appears to fall again (15%) at doses > 10 MU/day (Horoszewicz and Murphy 1989). These data are not randomised and must be interpreted with caution. The dose of 9–10 MU/day three times a week has become the standard regimen, partly for practical reasons and because of an acceptable balance between efficacy and toxicity.

The duration of INFα therapy for advanced RCC is an unresolved issue. The time taken to respond to interferon varies greatly. Most patients who respond to INFα treatment will have done so by 3–4 months. Occasionally responses can occur as late as 6–9 months after starting treatment, although not in patients who initially show progression during INFα treatment. There are no data from randomised controlled trials on the optimal duration of INFα therapy for patients who respond or for those who have stable disease. A common practice is to continue treatment indefinitely, provided there is no disease progression or significant toxicity.

The side effects of IFNα are very dose dependent and these include: tiredness, flu-like symptoms such as fever and shivering, loss of appetite, nausea and depression. They are most prominent during the first days of treatment and generally the patients feel better within 1–2 weeks. Furthermore, toxicity is usually very short-lived after cessation of the therapy. This last fact is important to point out to patients who are unsure about commencing treatment.

Interleukin-2

A second group of cytokines that has been found to be active in RCC is the interleukins, especially interleukin-2 (IL2). The protein IL2 is produced by activated T lymphocytes and it is a lymphocyte growth factor. It is required for proliferation and differentiation of naive T cells into activated effector T cells. It is thought that its anti-tumour activity is mediated by stimulation of an anti-tumour T-cell response rather than by direct anti-proliferative activity. This indirect anti-tumour effect is the reason why in early trials adoptive therapy used autologous lymphocytes (lymphokine-activated killer cells or LAK) administered together with IL2.

In the 1980s Rosenberg et al. (1985) reported an objective tumour response (partial response [PR] + complete response [CR]) in 11 of 25 (44%) patients with solid tumours (RCC, melanoma, colon cancer) who were treated with high-dose intravenous IL2 and LAK cells. Later, randomised trials (Rosenberg et al. 1993; Law et al. 1995) showed that anti-tumour activity in terms of response rate and survival were similar for patients treated with high-dose IL2 with or without LAK cells. In these more recent trials, the overall response rate for single-agent high-dose IL2 was much lower (10–30%) than initially reported. Fyfe and co-workers (1995) reported on 255 patients with metastatic RCC treated in this way. The overall response rate was 15%; however, complete remissions occurred in as many as 17 (7%) patients. The most significant finding in this study was that some of these complete responses were durable. An update of these data reported that the median response duration for patients who achieved CR was not reached after an observation time of more than 5 years, but is at least 80 months with 13 patients being alive and in complete remission more than 5 years after IL2 treatment. (Fisher et al. 2000). These data suggest that there is a group of long-term survivors who may even be regarded as cured after high-dose IL2 treatment. However, these data are not based on randomised controlled trials and the number of patients who have such a striking benefit is at best small.

The toxicity of high-dose intravenous IL2 regimens is of major concern. Flu-like symptoms, fever and chills are frequent, and a capillary leak syndrome resulting in severe hypotension and fluid retention, particularly pulmonary oedema, causes high morbidity. In the report of Fyfe and colleagues (1995) 10 (4%) patients died as a result of adverse events. Supportive measures, including vasopressor support on intensive care units, have reduced treatment-related mortality when IL2 is delivered in high doses by intravenous bolus injections to less than 1% in recent years, but toxicity remains a major problem with this treatment schedule. Other schedules and routes of administration have been investigated. Continuous as opposed to bolus intravenous infusion (West et al. 1987) of high-dose IL2 was associated with fewer and less severe adverse events, with similar response rates being obtained. However, this schedule still requires inpatient management.

Atzpodien and his group (1990) performed several trials using subcutaneous IL2 (in combination with INFα) and they found similar response rates with significantly less toxicity. Furthermore, these patients could be treated as outpatients. In 35 patients treated with subcutaneous IL2 and INFα, the main side effects were local inflammation at the injection site, fever and chills, mild hypotension, nausea and anorexia (Atzpodien et al. 1990). However, there are currently no data on whether or not long-term remissions are seen after subcutaneous IL2, in the same way as there are with high-dose bolus intravenous IL2.

The optimum dose schedule and duration of IL2 therapy remain uncertain. In a randomised prospective trial of 125 patients (Yang et al. 1994), treatment consisted of low-dose IL2 (72 000 IU/kg as intravenous bolus every 8 hours to a maximum of 15 doses, repeated after 7–10 days), one-tenth of the dose administered to the control group who received a standard high-dose intravenous bolus IL2 (720 000 IU/kg every 8 hours according to the same schedule). Lissoni et al. used a different schedule of low dose IL2 (3 million IU twice daily subcutaneously for 5 days per week, for six consecutive weeks in patients with metastatic RCC. They report survival rates of 50% at 10 years which was associated with patients who achieved response or stable disease on therapy (Lissoni et al. 2002).

Toxicity in terms of thrombocytopenia, malaise and hypotension was significantly lower in the low-dose group. Only 3% of treatment courses with low-dose IL2 prompted vasopressor support, as opposed to 52% of treatment courses with high-dose IL2, and response rates were similar in both groups (15% vs 20%) (Yang et al. 1994).

Most patients who respond to IL2 treatment show evidence of tumour regression as early as the first or second cycle (Lindsey et al. 2000) and, although the optimal treatment duration is not determined yet, currently most investigators would stop treatment if no objective response were observed after two cycles. In responders, treatment is continued until a complete remission is achieved or until IL2 intolerance develops.

IL2 and IFNα

Following the recognition that both IL2 and INFα had activity in the treatment of advanced RCC, the question arose as to whether combining these two agents would be beneficial. Phase II trials showed promising results, e.g. in a large multi-institutional study (Atzpodien et al. 1993a), the response rate was 19% with 4% complete remissions in 134 treated patients, using an outpatient subcutaneous combination regimen. In 1993, however, a randomised trial by Atkins et al. (1993) failed to show an advantage of adding IFNα (3 MU/m^2 every 8 hours i.v. on days 1–5 and 15–19) to high-dose bolus intravenous IL2.

A French collaborative group chose a different regimen for the combination of IL2 and IFNα as one of the treatments in a three-arm randomised trial (Negrier et al. 1998). They randomised 425 patients to receive: single agent IL2 administered as a 5-day continuous intravenous infusion at a dose of 18 MU/m^2 per day, repeated six times with 3-week intervals (138 patients, group 1); subcutaneous single agent IFNα at a dose of 18 MU three times a week for 23 weeks (147 patients, group 2); or the same IL2 treatment as group 1 but, in addition, IFNα at a dose of 6 MU three times per week during the IL2 cycles (140 patients, group 3). Response rates were 6.5%, 7.5% and 18.6% ($p < 0.001$) for the groups receiving IL2, IFNα and IL2 + IFNα, respectively. At 1 year, the event-free survival was still significantly higher for combination therapy (20%) than for single agent treatment (IL2 15%, IFNα 12%, $p = 0.01$), but there was no significant difference in overall survival among the three groups.

The same collaborative group also addressed the question of cross-resistance between IL2 and IFNα. They showed clearly (Escudier et al. 1999) that, if patients progress on IFNα or IL2 treatment, they are very unlikely to respond to the other cytokine. In fact, even if there was an initial response to first-line IFNα or IL2, a response to second-line therapy with the other cytokine after relapse/progression was very rare: only 4 of 113 patients responded to crossover treatment. Other investigators, however, document different results and have concluded that IL2 subcutaneous therapy alone can be an effective and well tolerated treatment in advanced RCC patients progressed under IFNα therapy (see Lissoni et al. 1992; Bordin et al. 2000).

Biochemotherapy
IL2/IFNα/5FU

RCC is resistant to most chemotherapeutic agents, although vinblastine and 5-fluorouracil (5FU) have some modest activity. The suggestion that cytokine treatment can enhance chemotherapeutic cytotoxicity is supported by early clinical trials. In 1993 Atzpodien and co-workers (1993b) treated 34 patients with advanced RCC with a combination therapy of IL2, IFNα and 5FU. Treatment consisted of 8 weeks of subcutaneous IFNα (6–9 MU/m^2 one to three times weekly) combined sequentially with subcutaneous IL2 (5–20 MU/m^2 three times weekly) for 4 weeks, and then 5FU (750 mg/m^2 intravenous bolus weekly) for 4 weeks. The overall response rate to this regimen was 49%, with 11% of the patients achieving a complete remission.

These encouraging results prompted several phase II studies testing the combination of these three drugs. In 1997 Bukowski summarised seven trials with a total of 262 patients: the overall response rate ranged from 10% to 39% with a mean of 32%, and complete remissions were observed in 0–16% of patients. These trials all had small numbers of patients and differed considerably with regard to the schedules used.

There is one randomised trial (Atzpodien et al. 2001) comparing IL2/IFNα/5FU biochemotherapy to hormonal treatment with tamoxifen. A total of 78 patients with advanced RCC were treated and the objective response rate in the biochemotherapy group was 39% as opposed to 0% in the tamoxifen group. Biochemotherapy was administered according to the schedule in Table 9.1.

Table 9.1

Weeks 1 and 4	IFNα (subcutaneous)	6 MU/m^2 per day	Day 1
	IL2 (subcutaneous)	10 MU/m^2 twice daily	Days 3, 4, 5
Weeks 2 and 3	IFNα (subcutaneous)	6 MU/ m^2 per day	Days 1, 3, 5
	IL2 (subcutaneous)	5 MU/ m^2 per day	Days 1, 3, 5
Weeks 5–8	IFNα (subcutaneous)	9 MU/ m^2 per day	Days 1, 3, 5
	5FU intravenous bolus	1000 mg/m^2 weekly	

The most remarkable observation was a significant survival benefit: the overall survival of patients treated with IL2/IFNα/5FU was 24 months, whereas the overall survival in the tamoxifen group was 13 months ($p = 0.0325$).

The role of 5FU in combination with IL2 and IFNα was addressed in another randomised trial with 131 patients (Negrier et al. 2000). The biochemotherapy regimen was different from that chosen by Atzpodien's group (above) (Table 9.2).

Table 9.2

Weeks 1, 3, 5, 7 (both arms)	IFNα (subcutaneous)	6 MU/day	Days 1, 3, 5
	IL2 (subcutaneous)	9 MU/day	Days 1–6
Weeks 1 and 5 (arm B) (continuous intravenous infusion)	5FU	600 mg/m^2 per day	Days 1–5

The patients in the control arm of this trial were treated with IL2 and IFNα without 5FU. Response rates in both groups were lower than expected, being 1% in the IL2/IFNα group and 8% in the IL2/IFNα/5FU group. Survival at one year was equal in both groups (53% vs 52%).

The reason for these conflicting results from different randomised studies is not fully understood, but the different treatment schedules probably explain some of the inconsistencies. In summary, the role of IL2/IFNα/5FU biochemotherapy is not yet determined.

IFNα/vinblastine

Vinblastine is known to have moderate activity in the treatment of RCC. Its combination with immunotherapy has not been as extensively studied as for 5FU, but three randomised trials have been published that have examined vinblastine-based biochemotherapy. In the first, 178 patients with metastatic RCC (Fossa et al. 1992) were treated with subcutaneous IFNα (18 MU/day three times a week) with or without vinblastine (0.1 mg/kg i.v. once every 3 weeks). The overall response rate in the combination therapy arm was 24% compared with 11% in the IFN single-agent arm. However, this increase in response rate did not translate into prolonged survival.

The other two studies comparing IFNα plus vinblastine to either vinblastine alone (Pyrhonen et al. 1999) or medroxyprogesterone acetate (Kriegmair et al. 1995) are discussed in the section on randomised controlled trials for 'immunotherapy versus non-immunotherapy'.

IFNα/retinoic acid

Retinoic acid has also been investigated as a possible agent to improve efficacy of IFNα treatment and response rates in phase II trials range from 3% to 30% (Escudier et al. 1998; Motzer et al. 1995; Stadler et al. 1998). In a large randomised trial of 284 patients (Motzer et al. 2000), the response rate and survival were not significantly different between the patients treated with IFNα plus retinoic acid and those who received IFNα alone.

IL2/IFNα/5FU±retinoic acid vs IFNα+vinblastine

A randomised trial comparing the role of different immunotherapy/chemotherapy combinations was published recently by the Atzpodien Group (Atzpodien et al. 2004). They randomized patients in three arms: Arm A (sc INFα2α + sc IL2 + iv 5FU), Arm B (Arm A + oral cis retinoic acid) and Arm C (sc INFα2α + iv vinblastine) with objective response rates of 31%, 26% and 20% respectively. Arm B, but not Arm A, showed a significantly improved progression free survival compared with Arm C. Both Arms A and B showed a significantly improved overall survival compared with Arm C. All three Arms were moderately or well tolerated, reinforcing the safety and improved efficacy of subcutaneous IL2 plus subcutaneous IFNα2α–based immunotherapies.

Randomised controlled trials of immunotherapy versus non-immunotherapy

There are many non-randomised trials of immunotherapy in RCC and only a few phase III studies. Some of these randomised trials have been mentioned above (Fossa et al. 1992; Negrier et al. 1998, 2000; Motzer et al. 2000; Atzpodien et al. 2001), but in this chapter we collate all those phase III studies that compare immunotherapy with a non-immunotherapy approach. All such studies use IFNα and there are no prospective randomised trials comparing IL2 without IFNα to a non-immunotherapy regimen or placebo. Six randomised controlled trials compare immunotherapy to a control and also report on survival and they are summarised below and in Table 9.3.

Henriksson and colleagues (1998) compared a combination immunotherapy (IFNα/IL2/tamoxifen) to tamoxifen monotherapy. The primary endpoint was survival and response rates for the 128 treated patients were therefore only partially reported. There was no difference in overall survival between the two groups.

Table 9.3 Randomised trials of regimens including IFNa versus control in patients with metastatic RCC

Reference	n	Treatment	Response rate (%)	Survival (median, months)
Steineck et al. (1990)	60	IFNα vs MPA	6 3	NS
Kriegmair et al. (1995)	76	IFNα + Vlb vs MPA	20.5 0	NS
Henriksson et al. (1998)	128	IFNα + IL2 + Tam vs Tam	– –	NS
MRC (1999)	335	IFNα vs MPA	13 7	8.5 6 (p = 0.017)
Pyrhonen et al. (1999)	160	IFNα + Vlb vs Vlb	16.5 2.5	16.9 9.5 (p = 0.0049)
Atzpodien et al. (2001)	78	IFNα + IL2 + 5FU vs Tam	39 0	24 13 (p = 0.0325)

IFN, interferon; IL2, interleukin-2; 5FU, 5-fluorouracil; MPA, medroxyprogesterone acetate; NS, difference not statistically significant; Tam, tamoxifen; Vlb, vinblastine.

Four randomised trials use IFNα as the sole cytokine in the immunotherapy arm:

- Steineck and co-workers (1990) treated 60 patients either with IFNα or medroxyprogesterone acetate (MPA) and there were only two responders in the IFN group and one patient with partial remission in the MPA group. No survival difference was observed. However, in this small trial 15 of 30 patients allocated to MPA crossed over to IFNα after MPA treatment.
- Kriegmair et al. (1995) published data on 76 patients treated with IFNα plus vinblastine or single agent MPA. The response rate in the immunotherapy group was 20.5%. and no remissions were reported in the patients treated with MPA; again this difference in response did not translate into a survival benefit.
- The two largest randomised trials were both published in 1999. In a Finnish trial (Pyrhonen et al. 1999), 160 patients with locally advanced or metastatic RCC received either subcutaneous IFNα (3 MU three times a week for 1 week, then 18 MU three times a week for 51 weeks) and vinblastine (0.1 mg/kg i.v. every 3 weeks for 1 year), or vinblastine (at the same dose) alone for 1 year or until disease progression. Overall response rates were 16.5% for patients treated with the combination and 2.5% for patients treated with vinblastine alone. Median survival was 67.6 weeks for patients on the IFNα/vinblastine arm and significantly longer than for patients on the vinblastine arm (37.8 weeks, p = 0.0049). Interestingly,

overall survival for the non-responding patients in the IFN-α/vinblastine group was significantly longer than for the non-responders in the vinblastine group. More than half of the patients (42 of 79 patients) in the immunotherapy arm reduced IFNα dose during the treatment period because of toxicity. However, there was no difference in survival for patients treated with 18 MU IFNα three times a week compared with those on a reduced dose of 9 MU.

- In the largest study that was performed in the UK (Medical Research Council Renal Cancer Collaborators 1999), 335 patients were randomised to receive either IFNα (10 MU s.c. three times a week for 12 weeks) or MPA (300 mg/day p.o. for 12 weeks). The overall response rate at 6 months was 13% for the patients in the IFN group and 7% for those receiving MPA. Median survival in the IFNα group was 8 months, which is 2.5 months (10 weeks) longer than for the MPA group (6 months), and this was statistically significant ($p = 0.017$). Survival at 1 year was 43% for the IFNα patients and 31% for the MPA patients. It is of note that the protocol stated that the treatment period was only 3 months in this study compared with 12 months of treatment in the other randomised study, which demonstrated a survival advantage for IFNα therapy. However, it is known that a number of responding patients continued with their treatment.

  At 4 weeks of treatment, patients receiving IFNα reported more side effects than the control group, including tiredness (73% of patients receiving IFN), lack of appetite (54%), nausea (28%), shivering (22%) and dry mouth (38%). At 12 weeks a larger proportion of IFNα patients reported moderate-to-severe lack of appetite (39% compared with 8% of patients on MPA), although a larger percentage of patients in the MPA group reported heartburn (33% compared with 8% of patients on IFN). Dose reduction was necessary in 24% of patients on IFNα and in 7% of patients on MPA. At 6 months, there was no evidence of difference in any of the reported toxicity-related symptoms between groups. In summary, IFNα treatment at a dose of 10 MU s.c. three times a week was relatively well tolerated after the initial side effects subsided.

In the recently published study of Atzpodien et al. (2001) on 78 patients, the survival benefit for patients treated with an outpatient schedule of IFNα/IL2/5FU was significant, with a median survival of 24 months compared with 13 months ($p = 0.0325$) for patients treated with tamoxifen.

Survival benefit of IFNα treatment: Cochrane Review

An extensive review on all randomised trials on immunotherapy for advanced RCC has been published in the Cochrane Library (Coppin et al. 2000). Forty-two randomised trials involving 4216 patients were considered. The primary question was whether immunotherapy in patients with advanced RCC conferred survival benefit. There were no studies that directly examined whether single-agent high-dose IL2 treatment improves survival compared with other treatments. In contrast six trials (Steineck et al. 1990; Kriegmair et al. 1995; Lummen et al. 1996; Henriksson et al. 1998; Medical Research Council Renal Cancer Collaborators 1999; Pyrhonen et al. 1999) reported survival data for regimens that included IFNα compared to other alternatives. This meta-analysis confirms a survival benefit of IFNα treatment with an average median improvement of survival of 2.6 months. The pooled hazard ratio for survival of 0.78 (0.67–0.90) indicates that the treatment effect persisted for 2 years from randomisation. There are no studies comparing IFNα to placebo or best supportive care, although the MPA control group virtually corresponds to a placebo control or 'best supportive care'. Data on quality of life during IFNα treatment are too sparse to explore any improvement in quality-adjusted life years.

Another important observation in this meta-analysis was that the difference in response rate between treatment arms correlated significantly with differences in survival. This suggests that response may be a surrogate endpoint for survival.

The recently published study of Atzpodien et al. (2001) comparing IFNα/IL2/5FU with tamoxifen is not yet included in the Cochrane Review but will further increase the evidence for a survival benefit with IFNα treatment.

Factors that influence outcome

The natural history of RCC varies considerably between patients and it can be influenced by immunotherapy only in a relatively small proportion of patients. A number of studies have identified prognostic factors for response to immunotherapy and for survival (Palmer et al. 1992; Jones et al. 1993; Fossa et al. 1995; Motzer et al. 1999).

The most important prognostic factor for survival is performance status. Motzer et al. (1999) found five independent pre-treatment risk factors for patients with metastatic RCC in a multivariate analysis of 670 patients who were treated with chemo- or immunotherapy: Karnofsky performance status < 80%, absence of prior nephrectomy, lactate dehydrogenase > 1.5 times the upper limit of normal, anaemia and corrected serum calcium > 10 mg/dl. The median survival time of patients in three distinct risk groups featuring none, one to two or three and more risk factors was 20, 10 and 4 months, respectively ($p < 0.0001$).

In 1992 Palmer et al. identified prognostic factors for survival in patients treated with IL2 (compare Table 9.4) and two large case–control studies confirmed the same prognostic factors for patients treated with IFNα (Fossa et al. 1995) or IL2 (Jones et al. 1993).

Two hundred and thirty-one patients with advanced RCC treated with IFN-based immunotherapy were compared with 327 control patients treated with chemotherapy from the Eastern Cooperative Oncology Group (ECOG) database by Fossa and co-workers (1995). Similarly, Jones et al. (1993) compared 327 patients receiving high-dose continuous intravenous infusion IL2 treatment with 390 patients from the ECOG database. Both trials report performance status 0, time between diagnosis and

Table 9.4 Prognostic factors for survival for patients with metastatic RCC treated with immunotherapy

Performance status (Palmer et al. 1992; Jones et al. 1993; Fossa et al. 1995; Motzer et al. 1999)

Nephrectomy (Flanigan et al. 2000; Mickisch et al. 2001)

Interval between diagnosis and metastasis (Palmer et al. 1992; Jones et al. 1993; Fossa et al. 1995)

Number of metastatic sites (Palmer et al. 1992; Jones et al. 1993; Fossa et al. 1995)

treatment > 24 months and a single site of metastasis as being good prognostic factors in terms of survival after immunotherapy. In the good prognostic group of patients with two or more of the above-mentioned features, the median survival of the patients treated with IFNα or IL2 was 23.3 months and 20.4 months, respectively, and significantly longer than the median survival of the patients in the chemotherapy control groups, being 11.4 months ($p < 0.001$) and 12.6 months ($p < 0.0001$) respectively.

There has in the past been considerable debate on the role of nephrectomy in metastatic RCC. Recently, two studies (Flanigan et al. 2000; Mickisch et al. 2001) have clearly shown that patients with metastatic RCC with a good performance status who are treated with IFNα lived significantly longer if they have a nephrectomy before starting their immunotherapy. The median survivals in the groups undergoing nephrectomy followed by immunotherapy were 12.5 months and 17 months in these two trials compared with 8.1 months and 7 months for the patients who did not undergo nephrectomy. Immunotherapy consisted of subcutaneous IFNα 5 MU/m^2 three times a week for 1 year and the response rates were not significantly different between the two study arms. In summary, because of the results of these two trials, nephrectomy is now recommended for patients with metastatic RCC, provided that their performance status is good.

Future strategies in the treatment of advanced RCC

The median survival for patients with metastatic RCC is still short, being 10–15 months in most recent studies, and new treatment strategies are needed.

Biochemotherapy with IL2, IFNα and 5FU has shown promising initial results and therefore merits further investigation. This is currently done in an MRC trial in the UK (REO4), comparing this biochemotherapy regimen with single agent IFNα in patients with metastatic disease, and the EORTC and CRC are comparing IFNα/IL2/5FU with observation only in the adjuvant setting. The EORTC 30955 adjuvant triple study has now closed as a European study but it is hoped that it will continue in the UK under a new lead UK investigator. The new re-named study (HYDRA) ("Helping You Decrease your Recurrence After nephrectomy") will be led by the Beaston Oncology Centre at Glasgow, UK and it is anticipated that the trial will re-start within UK study centres in late 2004.

The pegylated form of interferon could possibly reduce toxicity of IFNα treatment and facilitate its administration, and this new formulation also merits investigation.

Another area of great interest is that of different immunisation strategies. As with melanoma, RCC is an immunogenic tumour and initially promising results need to be confirmed by carefully designed prospective studies.

One of the modes of action of IFNα is inhibition of angiogenesis. Many new angiogenesis inhibitors are currently being investigated. Thalidomide, which has anti-angiogenic activity among a number of other actions, has shown activity in advanced RCC in phase II trials conducted at the Royal Marsden Hospital with response rates of 10–27% (Eisen et al. 2000; Stebbing et al. 2001). This treatment has the advantage of its good tolerability and easy administration and could be an option for patients who are not fit enough for immunotherapy. Currently, a randomised trial comparing thalidomide with MPA for patients with advanced RCC who are not suitable for immunotherapy is ongoing. Other angiogenesis inhibitors, including direct blockers of the vascular endothelial growth factor (VEGF) receptor, are in early clinical trials.

Conclusions

A proportion of patients with metastatic RCC gain a survival benefit from immunotherapy. Interpretation of the literature on immunotherapy in RCC is difficult because most of the studies are small, non-randomised and vary considerably in patient selection and the treatment regimens given. However, it is clear that IFNα treatment has been shown to confer a survival benefit to patients with advanced RCC. This was demonstrated in two randomised controlled studies (Medical Research Council Renal Cancer Collaborators 1999; Pyrhonen et al. 1999) and confirmed by the Cochrane Review (Coppin et al. 2000). Therefore, the control arm in future randomised studies for treatment of metastatic RCC should be IFNα. Doses of 5–10 MU/day seem to be most effective. Optimal treatment duration has not been established yet.

Responses to high-dose IL2 treatment are reported to be of very long duration in a small proportion of patients (Fisher et al. 2000). However, there are no randomised data to show that this treatment confers a survival advantage and toxicity of high-dose IL2 therapy is considerable.

Biochemotherapy, particularly the combination of IL2, IFNα and 5FU, has been shown to be active in metastatic RCC but needs further investigation in randomised trials.

Radical nephrectomy before immunotherapy is recommended in patients with metastatic RCC and good performance status, based on the significant survival benefit seen in two randomised trials (Flanigan et al. 2000; Mickisch et al. 2001).

Performance status is the most important prognostic factor for survival in metastatic RCC, and patients should be carefully assessed for all the relevant prognostic factors before starting immunotherapy.

References

Atkins MB, Sparano J, Fisher RI et al. (1993) Randomized phase II trial of high-dose interleukin-2 either alone or in combination with interferon alfa-2b in advanced renal cell carcinoma. *Journal of Clinical Oncology* **11**: 661–670.

Atzpodien, J, Korfer, A, Franks, CR, Poliwoda, H, Kirchner, H (1990) Home therapy with recombinant interleukin-2 and interferon-alpha 2b in advanced human malignancies. *The Lancet* **335**: 1509–1512.

Atzpodien J, Kirchner H, de Mulder P et al. (1993a) Subcutaneous recombinant interleukin-2 and alpha-interferon in patients with advanced renal cell carcinoma: results of a multicenter Phase II Study. *Cancer Biotherapy* **8**: 289–300.

Atzpodien J, Kirchner H, Hanninen EL, Deckert M, Fenner M, Poliwoda H (1993b) Interleukin-2 in combination with interferon-alpha and 5-fluorouracil for metastatic renal cell cancer. *European Journal of Cancer* **29A**: S6–S8.

Atzpodien J, Kirchner H, Illiger HJ et al. (2001) IL-2 in combination with IFN- alpha and 5-FU versus tamoxifen in metastatic renal cell carcinoma: long-term results of a controlled randomized clinical trial. *British Journal of Cancer* **85**: 1130–1136.

Atzpodien J, Kirchner H, Jonas U et al. (2004) Interleukin-2- and Interferon Alfa-2a-based immunochemotherapy in advanced renal cell carcinoma: a prospectively randomised trial of the German Cooperative Renal Carcinoma Chemoimmunotherapy Group (DGCIN). *Journal of Clinical Oncology* **22**: 1188–1194.

Bordin V, Giani L, Meregalli S et al. (2000) Five year survival results of subcutaneous low-dose immunotherapy with Interleukin-2 alone in metastatic renal cell cancer patients. *Urologia Internationalis* **64**: 3–8.

Bukowski RM (1997) Natural history and therapy of metastatic renal cell carcinoma: the role of interleukin-2. *Cancer* **80**: 1198–1220.

Cancer Research Campaign (1999) The CRC CancerStats (www.crc.org.uk)

Casali M, Marcellini M, Casali A, Giuntini T, Galante E, Ferrone C (2001) Gemcitabine in pre-treated advanced renal carcinoma: a feasibility study. *Journal of Experimental Clinical Cancer Research* **20**: **195**–8.

Coppin, C Porzsolt F, Kumpf J, Coldman A, Wilt T (2000) Immunotherapy for advanced renal cell cancer. *Cochrane Database System Rev*iew CD001425.

Eisen T, Boshoff C, Mak I et al. (2000) Continuous low dose thalidomide: a phase II study in advanced melanoma, renal cell, ovarian and breast cancer. *British Journal of Cancer* **82**: 812–817.

Escudier B, Ravaud A, Berton D, Chevreau C, Douillard JY, Dietrich PY (1998) Phase II study of interferon-alpha and all-trans retinoic acid in metastatic renal cell carcinoma. *Journal of Immunotherapy* **21**: 62–64.

Escudier B, Chevreau C, Lasset C et al. (1999) Cytokines in metastatic renal cell carcinoma: is it useful to switch to interleukin-2 or interferon after failure of a first treatment? Groupe Francais d'Immunotherapie. *Journal of Clinical Oncology* **17**: 2039–2043.

Fisher RI, Rosenberg SA, Fyfe G (2000) Long-term survival update for high-dose recombinant interleukin-2 in patients with renal cell carcinoma. *Cancer Journal of the Scientific American* **6**: S55–S57.

Flanigan R, Blumenstein B, Salmon S (2000) Cytoreductive tumornephrectomy in metastatic renal cancer: the results of Southwest Oncology Group Trial 8949. *Journal of Urology* **163**: 685 (abstract).

Fossa SD, Martinelli G, Otto U et al. (1992) Recombinant interferon alfa-2a with or without vinblastine in metastatic renal cell carcinoma: results of a European multi-center phase III study. *Annals of Oncology* **3**: 301–305.

Fossa S, Jones M, Johnson P et al. (1995) Interferon-alpha and survival in renal cell cancer. *British Journal of Urology* **76**: 286–290.

Fyfe G, Fisher RI, Rosenberg SA, Sznol M, Parkinson DR, Louie AC (1995) Results of treatment of 255 patients with metastatic renal cell carcinoma who received high-dose recombinant interleukin-2 therapy. *Journal of Clinical Oncology* **13**: 688–696.

Gleave ME, Elhilali M, Fradet Y et al. (1998) Interferon gamma-1b compared with placebo in metastatic renal-cell carcinoma. Canadian Urologic Oncology Group. *New England Journal of Medicine* **338**: 1265–1271.

Henriksson R, Nilsson S, Colleen S et al. (1998) Survival in renal cell carcinoma-a randomized evaluation of tamoxifen vs interleukin 2, alpha-interferon (leucocyte) and tamoxifen. *British Journal of Cancer* **77**: 1311–1317.

Horoszewicz JS, Murphy GP (1989) An assessment of the current use of human interferons in therapy of urological cancers. *Journal of Urology* **142**: 1173–1180.

Jones M, Philip T, Palmer P et al. (1993) The impact of interleukin-2 on survival in renal cancer: a multivariate analysis. *Cancer Biotherapy* **8**: 275–288.

Kriegmair M, Oberneder R, Hofstetter A (1995) Interferon alfa and vinblastine versus medroxyprogesterone acetate in the treatment of metastatic renal cell carcinoma. *Urology* **45**: 758–762.

Law TM, Motzer RJ, Mazumdar M et al. (1995) Phase III randomized trial of interleukin-2 with or without lymphokine-activated killer cells in the treatment of patients with advanced renal cell carcinoma. *Cancer* **76**: 824–832.

Lindsey KR, Rosenberg SA, Sherry R.M. (2000) Impact of the number of treatment courses on the clinical response of patients who receive high-dose bolus interleukin-2. *Journal of Clinical Oncology* **18**: 1954–1959.

Lissoni P, Barni S, Ardizzoia A et al. (1992) Second line therapy with low dose subcutaneous interleukin-2 alone in advanced renal cancer patients resistant to interferon-alpha. *European Journal of Cancer* **28**: 92–96.

Lissoni P, Bordin V, Vaghi M et al. (2002) Ten year survival results in metastatic renal cell cancer patients treated with monoimmunotherapy with subcutaneous low-dose Interleukin-2. *Anticancer Research* **22**: 1061–1064.

Lummen G, Goepel M, Mollhoff S, Hinke A, Otto T, Rubben H (1996) Phase II study of interferon-gamma versus interleukin-2 and interferon-alpha 2b in metastatic renal cell carcinoma. *Journal of Urology* **155**: 455–458.

Medical Research Council Renal Cancer Collaborators (1999) Interferon-alpha and survival in metastatic renal carcinoma: early results of a randomised controlled trial. Medical Research Council Renal Cancer Collaborators. *The Lancet* **353**: 14–17.

Mickisch G, Garin A, van Poppel H, de Prijck L, Sylvester R, Members of the European Organisation for Research and Treatment of Cancer (EORTC) Genitourinary Group (2001) Radical nephrectomy plus interferon-alfa-based immunotherapy compared with interferon alfa alone in metastatic renal-cell carcinoma: a randomised trial. *The Lancet* **358**: 966–970.

Motzer RJ, Schwartz L, Law TM et al. (1995) Interferon alfa-2a and 13-cis-retinoic acid in renal cell carcinoma: antitumor activity in a phase II trial and interactions in vitro. *Journal of Clinical Oncology* **13**: 1950–1957.

Motzer RJ, Mazumdar M, Bacik J, Berg W, Amsterdam A, Ferrara J (1999) Survival and prognostic stratification of 670 patients with advanced renal cell carcinoma. *Journal of Clinical Oncology* **17**: 2530–2540.

Motzer RJ, Murphy BA, Bacik J et al. (2000) Phase III trial of interferon alfa-2a with or without 13-cis-retinoic acid for patients with advanced renal cell carcinoma. *Journal of Clinical Oncology* **18**: 2972–2980.

Negrier S, Escudier B, Lasset C et al. (1998) Recombinant human interleukin-2, recombinant human interferon alfa-2a, or both in metastatic renal-cell carcinoma Groupe Français d'Immunotherapie. *New England Journal of Medicine* **338**: 1272–1278.

Negrier S, Caty A, Lesimple T et al. (2000) Treatment of patients with metastatic renal carcinoma with a combination of subcutaneous interleukin-2 and interferon alfa with or without fluorouracil Groupe Francais d'Immunotherapie, Federation Nationale des Centres de Lutte Contre le Cancer. *Journal of Clinical Oncology* **18**: 4009–4015.

Palmer PA, Vinke J, Philip T et al. (1992) Prognostic factors for survival in patients with advanced renal cell carcinoma treated with recombinant interleukin-2. *Annals of Oncology* **3**: 475–480.

Pyrhonen S, Salminen E, Ruutu M et al. (1999) Prospective randomized trial of interferon alfa-2a plus vinblastine versus vinblastine alone in patients with advanced renal cell cancer. *Journal of Clinical Oncology* **17**: 2859–2867.

Rosenberg SA, Lotze MT, Muul LM et al. (1985) Observations on the systemic administration of autologous lymphokine-activated killer cells and recombinant interleukin-2 to patients with metastatic cancer. *New England Journal of Medicine* **313**: 1485–1492.

Rosenberg SA, Lotze MT, Yang JC et al. (1993) Prospective randomized trial of high-dose interleukin-2 alone or in conjunction with lymphokine-activated killer cells for the treatment of patients with advanced cancer. *Journal of the National Cancer Institute* **85**: 622–632.

Stadler WM, Kuzel T, Dumas M, Vogelzang NJ (1998) Multicenter phase II trial of interleukin-2, interferon-alpha, and 13-cis-retinoic acid in patients with metastatic renal-cell carcinoma. *Journal of Clinical Oncology* **16**: 1820–1825.

Stebbing J, Benson C, Eisen T et al. (2001) The treatment of advanced renal cell cancer with high-dose oral thalidomide. *British Journal of Cancer* **85**: 953–958.

Steineck G, Strander H, Carbin BE et al. (1990) Recombinant leukocyte interferon alpha-2a and medroxyprogesterone in advanced renal cell carcinoma. A randomized trial. *Acta Oncologica* **29**: 155–162.

Webb A, Gore M (2000) The management of metastatic renal cell cancer. *UroOncology* **1**: 1–6.

Wenzel C, Schmidinger M, Locker G et al. (2001) Capecitabine in the treatment of metastatic renal cell carcinoma failing immunotherapy – the Vienna experience. *Proceedings of the American Society of Clinical Oncology* **20**: 196a (abstract 782).

West WH, Tauer KW, Yannelli JR et al. (1987) Constant-infusion recombinant interleukin-2 in adoptive immunotherapy of advanced cancer. *New England Journal of Medicine* **316**: 898–905.

Yang JC, Topalian SL, Parkinson D et al. (1994) Randomized comparison of high-dose and low-dose intravenous interleukin-2 for the therapy of metastatic renal cell carcinoma: an interim report. *Journal of Clinical Oncology* **12**: 1572–1576.

Chapter 10

Analysing current controversies on the utility of adjuvant therapy

Vincent J O'Neill and Paul A Vasey

Renal cell cancer accounts for approximately 3% of all adult solid tumours and is typically a disease of the fifth and sixth decades of life. Adequate surgical excision of non-metastatic tumours remains the only real possibility of cure. Many patients will experience relapse and up to 50% of patients present initially with regional or distal metastases. Almost 90% of patients with localised tumours survive for 5 years after diagnosis, whereas this falls to around 60% for those with regional disease and less than 10% for those with metastases.

The current standard surgical approach is removal of the kidney together with the adrenal and perirenal fat within the intact Gerota's fascia. A complete lymph node dissection, rather than removal of only visibly abnormal nodes, remains controversial. To date, there is no evidence of a survival benefit from lymphadenectomy. The technique does, however, provide valuable staging and prognostic information. Should lymphadenectomy be undertaken, a standard lumbar approach does not permit sufficient access to the whole area of the regional nodes, and a thoracoabdominal, midline or transverse abdominal incision is required. Ongoing issues in the management of renal cancer are summarised in Table 10.1.

Table 10.1 Issues in the treatment of renal cancer

Stage	Standard treatment	Outstanding issues
I	Nephrectomy	Surgical, e.g. nephron-sparing laparoscopic surgery
II	Nephrectomy	Role of lymphadenectomy Postoperative radiotherapy for compromised margins
III	Nephrectomy	Role of lymphadenectomy in N0 Postoperative radiotherapy for compromised margins Adjuvant systemic therapy
IV	Nephrectomy (selected patients)	Immunotherapy vs quality of life Combination immunotherapy vs monotherapy Chemoimmunotherapy Anti-angiogenesis agents

Adjuvant therapy after a definitive surgical procedure has become firmly established in the management of a number of adult solid tumours, and has demonstrable survival advantage in, for example, breast and colon cancer. For adjuvant treatments to have a place in the management of a disease, two criteria must be met: (1) the disease must have identifiable and reproducible risk factors for recurrence after curative local therapy; and (2) effective therapy must be available with clear anti-tumour activity as evidenced in the metastatic setting. The nature of these risk factors, their relative importance and the availability of effective anti-tumour agents in renal cancer are the subject of this review.

Risk factors for recurrent disease

Renal cell carcinoma (RCC) is well recognised as a tumour with an unpredictable but generally indolent course. Pathological stage remains the single most important prognostic factor. After surgery alone, 95% of Robson stage I patients (tumours confined to renal capsule) will be alive at 5 years. This figure falls with regional disease, e.g. node positivity, spread beyond Gerota's fascia and venous extension. As discussed elsewhere in this book, many physicians prefer the TNM classification of stage because it separates venous involvement from nodal invasion and quantifies each. On the basis of TNM stage, a T3a tumour has a much lower recurrence risk than a T3b or T3c (Table 10.2). In a study of 445 patients at the MD Anderson, T3a patients (locoregional) had a 5-year survival rate of 63% compared with T3b and T3c (involved renal vein) patients' survival rate of 37%. These patients could potentially be excluded from the group to whom adjuvant therapy is offered, because this relatively good outcome would require prospective studies to be very large indeed to define a clinically relevant outcome benefit.

Table 10.2 Comparison of Robson and TNM systems for staging of renal cell carcinoma

	Robson	TNM (1978)
Small tumour, minimal calyceal distortion (confined to renal capsule)	I	T1
Large tumour, calyceal distortion (confined to renal capsule)	I	T2
Tumour extension to perirenal fat or ipsilateral adrenal gland (confined by Gerota's fascia)	II	T3a
Renal vein involvement	IIIa	T3b
Renal vein and vena cava involvement	IIIa	T3c
Vena cava involvement above diaphragm	IIIa	T4b
Single ipsilateral node involved	IIIb	N1
Multiple regional, contralateral, or bilateral nodes involved	IIIb	N2
Fixed regional nodes	IIIb	N3
Juxtaregional nodes involved	IIIb	N4
Combination of IIIa and IIIb	IIIc	T3, 4 N1-4
Spread to contiguous organs except ipsilateral adrenal gland	IVa	T4a
Distant metastases	IVb	M1

Node-positive tumours generally have a worse prognosis than node-negative ones. Indeed, the 5-year survival rate for a patient with a single positive node is 20%, falling progressively as the number of positive regional node groups increases (Pizzocaro 1986). The role of lymphadenectomy in the surgical management of RCC is discussed elsewhere, but there is still no robust evidence that it confers a survival advantage, particularly in those without enlarged nodes at surgery. The technique does, however, have an important role in the proper staging of patients.

Haematogenous spread of RCC is the most frequent means of dissemination (Figures 10.1 and 10.2). Tumour extension into the renal vein has therefore traditionally been viewed as a poor prognostic factor. However, some studies have failed to show this correlation (Skinner et al. 1972; Selli et al. 1983) and it is possible that venous extension is not an independent prognostic indicator but is dependent on other factors. On the other hand, microvascular invasion is an important predictor of disease relapse after radical nephrectomy. In a recent study of 180 patients, microscopic vascular invasion without capsular invasion or lymph node positivity was associated with a recurrence rate of 45% at 1 year (van Poppel et al. 1997). The authors concluded that, in patients undergoing radical surgery for RCC without macroscopic invasion or positive lymph nodes, microscopic vascular invasion is the most important predicator of outcome. Extension of tumour into perirenal fat is likely to be associated with other poor prognostic markers, but independently increases the likelihood of positive lymph nodes at lymphadenectomy (Skinner et al. 1971). This makes it important as an independent risk factor in addition to lymph node positivity.

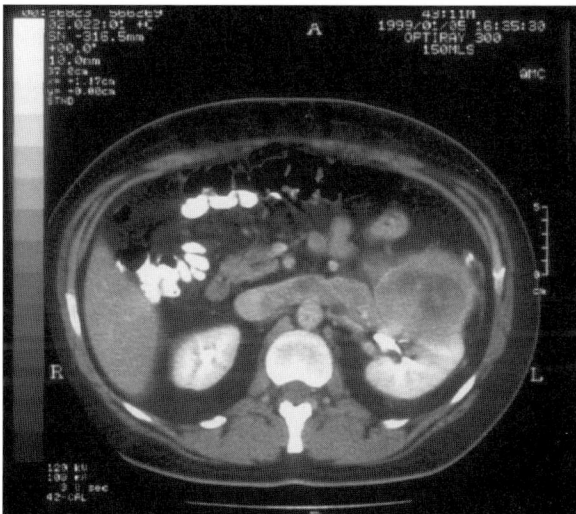

Figure 10.1 Renal carcinoma with renal vein involvement.

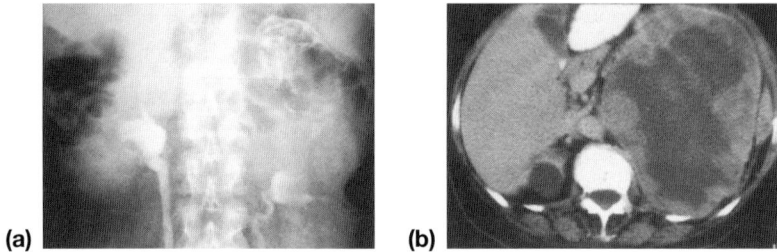

Figure 10.2 (a) Intravenous urogram, showing calcified left upper pole renal cancer with distorted calyceal pattern. (b) Large renal cancer with patent renal vein.

In summary, those factors predicting for tumour recurrence that may allow patients to be selected for adjuvant therapy are (1) positive nodes at lymphadenectomy, (2) extension of tumour into perinephric fat and (3) microscopic vascular invasion. Factors possibly predisposing to recurrence, but that are more likely to be interactive with other factors, include renal vein extension and tumour size.

Treatment modalities for the adjuvant setting

Hormone manipulation has been explored in the treatment of metastatic RCC. The presence of oestrogen and progestogen receptors on renal cancer cells has prompted the use of tamoxifen, megestrol acetate (Megace) and medroxyprogesterone acetate (Provera) in this setting. Unfortunately the response rates seen are less than 10% and, aside from the anti-anorectic effects of the progestogens, their use as cytotoxic agents is unjustified. Classic chemotherapeutic agents, used as single agents and in combination, likewise show a disappointing lack of activity in this tumour type (Vugrin 1987; Yagoda and Bander 1989). This may be a function of the very high expression of P-glycoprotein and similar mediators of multidrug resistance. To date, attempts to modulate multidrug resistance have failed to improve response rates for chemotherapy in this disease.

Renal cancer is a relatively radioresistant tumour type. Nevertheless, radiotherapy has a useful role in palliating symptoms from locoregional disease recurrence and skeletal metastases. Its role in the postoperative adjuvant setting is, however, controversial, and there are conflicting results from the few published studies.

Postoperative radiotherapy has been shown to be beneficial in three retrospective series (Table 10.3). In a study involving 240 patients, Rafla and Parikh (1984) claimed better local control and survival rates in patients receiving postoperative radiotherapy compared with nephrectomy alone (57 vs 37% overall survival rate at 5 years). However, the methodology was vague in that neither patient characteristics nor treatment regimens were well described. More recently, Stein and associates (1992) examined retrospectively 119 patients, 56 of whom had stage T3–4 tumours and underwent radiotherapy after surgery using computed tomography (CT) planning techniques. Local failure rates were 9% vs 22% in favour of treatment, and the 5-year overall survival rate was 50% vs 40%. Kao et al. (1994) reported similar results in T3–4 tumours again using CT planning, but patient numbers were small. Interestingly, no patient was reported to have experienced any complication secondary to radiotherapy in either of these two studies.

Table 10.3 Adjuvant postoperative radiotherapy studies: positive studies

Author	Patients	Treatment	5-year survival rate (%)	Comments
Rafla and Parikh (1984)	135	Nephrectomy	37	Retrospective, ?
	105	Nephrectomy + radiotherapy	57	patient selection
Stein et al. (1992)	63	Nephrectomy	40	Retrospective,
	56	Nephrectomy + radiotherapy	50	T2–4, CT planning
Kao et al. (1994)	12	Nephrectomy	62	Retrospective,
	12	Nephrectomy + radiotherapy	75	T3–4, CT planning

The two reported prospective studies of radiotherapy in this setting have not supported these positive findings (Table 10.4). Kjaer et al. (1987) randomised 65 patients with T2–3 disease either to receive or not to receive radiotherapy postoperatively. Although recurrence rates were no different in either arm, the 5-year survival rate in those receiving radiotherapy was 38%, compared with 63% in the group receiving surgery alone. In an earlier study, Finney and colleagues (1997) randomised 100 patients to surgery or surgery and radiotherapy with equivalent recurrence rates, but again inferior 5-year survival rates for the radiotherapy cohort (36% vs 47%). No stratification of patients by stage of disease was performed. Both these studies can be criticised on the grounds of inadequate patient selection and suboptimal radiation techniques, the latter reflected in the very high complication rates reported by Kjaer et al. (1987). Certainly, modern radiotherapy technique might be expected to be associated with fewer side effects and potentially better survival. However, other studies evaluating in a randomised manner the role of preoperative radiotherapy showed no advantage in local control for radiotherapy (Juusela et al. 1977; van der Werf-Messing et al. 1978).

Table 10.4 Adjuvant postoperative radiotherapy studies: negative studies

Author	Patients	Treatment	5-year survival rate (%)	Comments
Finney et al. (1973)	48	Nephrectomy	47	Randomised
	52	Nephrectomy + radiotherapy	36	No patient stratification
				> 20% radiotherapy complications
Kjaer et al. (1987)	33	Nephrectomy	63	Randomised
	32	Nephrectomy + radiotherapy	38	T2–3
				44% radiotherapy complications (19% fatal)

The pattern of disease relapse after 'curative' nephrectomy would be an important predictor of whether adjuvant locoregional therapy using radiotherapy might improve clinical outcome and overall survival. In fact, locoregional failure, including recurrence at the tumour bed and at the nephrectomy scar, is uncommon compared with metastatic relapse. In one series of 116 patients attending the Ottawa regional cancer centre with unilateral, non-metastatic RCC (Aref et al. 1997), 75 patients developed recurrences; 77% of these developed distant metastases, whereas only 10% experienced locoregional failure and a further 12% developed both locoregional and distal recurrence. From these data, one can conclude that the majority of patients who develop disease recurrence are likely to have occult metastases at the time of presentation. Such patients are therefore *unlikely* to benefit from adjuvant locoregional therapy.

Immunotherapy

Evidence that immunocompetence might be relevant in renal cancer has prompted the exploration of both specific and non-specific immunotherapies, with and without chemotherapy, in advanced and early disease. Specific emphasis has been placed on interferon (IFN) and interleukin-2 (IL2). In vitro models show that interferon has a direct anti-proliferative effect on tumour cells, and may also increase the expression of the major histocompatibility complex (MHC) antigen of tumour cells and activate macrophages, T lymphocytes and natural killer (NK) cells (Greiner et al. 1987). Most studies have provided evidence for modest but reproducible anti-tumour activity in advanced RCC. For interferon, the response rate (complete response [CR] + partial response [PR]) recorded from adequate trials (those with more than 20 evaluable patients and IFN doses exceeding 3 MIU/day) varies from 5% to 26%, with a mean of 17%. An overall response rate of 15% (median duration 54 months, range 3–104) was observed in a 255-patient database based on seven phase II studies with high-dose, bolus IL2 (Fisher et al. 1997). There were seven complete responders and the long duration of these led to FDA approval of this agent for use in the USA. Considerable improvement in IL2 toxicity can be achieved by administration by the subcutaneous route (e.g. Lissoni et al. 1992). Combining IFN and IL2 can be shown to improve response rates but does not appear to impact on survival in a recently reported randomised study (Negrier et al. 1998).

Adjuvant immunotherapy trials

In animal models, immunotherapeutic approaches were shown to be most effective in microscopic disease (Mule et al. 1986). Correspondingly, in patients with metastatic renal cancer, the highest response rates are generally seen in those with a low tumour burden, particularly with no brain or bone metastases. As we have active agents, the rationale for testing these in the adjuvant setting is clear.

To date, three randomised, prospective trials have examined the role of adjuvant immunotherapy in nephrectomised patients, two of which have appeared in abstract form only. None has shown a survival advantage for active treatment. Pizzocaro and colleagues (2001) have reported a multicentre, randomised trial comparing adjuvant IFNα with observation alone after radical nephrectomy in 247 patients with stage II and III disease. The 5-year overall survival and event-free survival were not significantly different in one group over the other. The authors did, however, point out a small possible advantage for patients with pN2/N3 disease, and recommended further investigation in this small subgroup.

The Delta-P study group similarly randomised 270 pT3/4N0/2M0 patients to adjuvant therapy with IFNα or observation alone following radical surgery. At 3 years, there was no difference in time to treatment failure or survival (Porsolt 1992). Lastly, Trump et al. (1996) reported an intergroup trial of lymphoblastoid IFN in 294 resected T3/4aN1–3 patients. At a median follow-up of 4.4 years, 56 patients in the observation group and 65 in the IFN group had developed recurrences.

Atzpodien reported a response rate of 31% in 32 patients with metastatic RCC, using a combination of IFN and IL2 subcutaneously (Atzpodien et al. 1993b), although a multicentre study found a lower response rate of 17% with this regimen. Using a combination of IFN, IL2 and 5-fluorouracil (5FU), a phase II study by the same author demonstrated an overall response rate of 48% (Atzpodien et al. 1993a). The treatment was administered to the patients as outpatients, and no grade IV toxicities were seen. In a report of a single centre experience with outpatient-based triple therapy involving 120 patients, an overall response rate of 39% was reported (Lopez Hanninen et al. 1996). Since then, a number of trials have confirmed the activity of this combination (median response rate 32%). However, many groups have failed to demonstrate these high response rates, and there are toxicity issues with this regimen that require experienced staff to manage.

Current status of adjuvant therapy for RCC

On the basis of current evidence, off-protocol adjuvant immunotherapy with IFN or IL2 is not appropriate for patients having had radical surgery for renal cancer. The Cancer Research Council (CRC) and the European Organisation for Research and Treatment of Cancer (EORTC) are running an international, multicentre trial evaluating IFN, IL and 5FU given by the Atzpodien schedule (Atzpodien et al. 1995) (Table 10.5) versus no treatment, in surgically treated renal cancer at high risk of recurrence. Although removal of clinically enlarged nodes is obligatory, lymph node dissection is optional. Eligible patients are those with: pathological stage T3b, T3c or T4; or any pT and nodal status N1 or N2; or any pT and microscopic positive margins; or the presence of any pT stage with microscopic vascular invasion. Randomisation between triple therapy and observation alone should take place within 8 weeks of surgery, and the trial aims to recruit 550 patients. It is designed to detect a 15% improvement in disease-free survival with type I ($\alpha = 0.05$). Currently, over 100 patients have been randomised and an interim analysis is planned. Problems with recruitment are, however, hampering this important study. Treatment costs and toxicity are considerable, raising issues of patient consent and centralised funding.

Table 10.5 The Atzpodien regimen (Atzpodien et al. 1995)

Week(s)	Day(s)	Interferon (MIU/m²)	Interleukin-2 (MIU/m²)	5-Fluorouracil (mg/m²)
1	1	6		
	3, 4, 5		10 twice daily	
2–3	1, 3, 5	6	5	
4	1	6		
	3, 4, 5		10 twice daily	
5–8	1	9		750
	3, 5	9		

Conclusion and future directions

Lack of supportive data from randomised trials for the routine use of adjuvant chemoimmunotherapy means that randomisation in the EORTC study 30955 should be strongly encouraged. In the meantime, a meta-analysis of the available data should be performed to allow a subgroup of patients to be identified who would potentially benefit from therapy. Novel agents, e.g. anti-angiogenics, may be useful if found to be associated with survival improvements in the metastatic setting.

References

Aref I, Bociek RG, Salhani D (1997) Is postoperative radiation for renal cell carcinoma justified? *Radiotherapy and Oncology* **43**: 155–157.

Atzpodien, Kirchner H, Hanninen EL, Deckert M, Fenner M, Poliwoda H (1993a) Interleukin-2 in combination with interferon-alpha and 5-fluorouracil for metastatic renal cell cancer. *European Journal of Cancer* 29A(suppl 5): S6–8.

Atzpodien, Kirchner H, de Mulder P et al. (1993b) Subcutaneous recombinant interleukin-2 and alpha-interferon in patients with advanced renal cell carcinoma: results of a multicenter Phase II Study. *Cancer Biotherapy* **8**: 289–300.

Atzpodien J, Lopez Hanninen E, Kirchner H et al. (1995) Multiinstitutional home-therapy trial of recombinant human interleukin-2 and interferon alfa-2 in progressive metastatic renal cell carcinoma. *Journal of Clinical Oncology* **13**: 497–501.

Finney R. (1973) The value of radiotherapy in the treatment of hypernephroma – a clinical trial. *British Journal of Urology* **45**: 258–269.

Fisher RJ, Rosenberg SA, Sznol M et al. (1997) High dose aldesleukin in renal cell carcinoma: long term survival update. *Cancer Journal of Scientific American* **3**(suppl 1): S70–S72.

Greiner JW, Guadagni F, Noguchi P et al. (1987) Recombinant interferon enhances monoclonal antibody-targeting of carcinoma lesions in vivo. *Science* **235**: 895–898.

Juusela H, Malmio K, Alfthan O, Oravisto KJ (1977) Preoperative radiotherapy in the treatment of renal adenocarcinoma. *Scandinavian Journal of Urology and Nephrology* **11**: 277–281.

Kao GD, Malkowicz SB, Whittington R, D'Amico AV, Wein AJ (1994) Locally advanced renal cell carcinoma: low complication rate and efficacy of postnephrectomy radiation therapy planned with CT. *Radiology* **193**: 725–730.

Kjaer M, Frederiksen PL, Engelholm SA (1987) Postoperative radiotherapy in stage II and III renal adenocarcinoma. A randomized trial by the Copenhagen Renal Cancer Study Group. *International Journal of Radiation Oncology, Biology and Physics* **13**: 665–672.

Lissoni P, Barni S, Ardizzoia A et al. (1992) Second line therapy with low-dose subcutaneous interleukin-2 alone in advanced renal cancer patients resistant to interferon-alpha. *European Journal of Cancer* **28**: 92–96.

Lopez Hanninen E, Kirchner H, Atzpodien J (1996) Interleukin-2 based home therapy of metastatic renal cell carcinoma: risks and benefits in 215 consecutive single institution patients. *Journal of Urology* **155**: 19–25.

Mule JJ, Ettinghausen SE, Spiess PJ, Shu S, Rosenberg SA (1986) Antitumor efficacy of lymphokine-activated killer cells and recombinant interleukin-2 in vivo: survival benefit and mechanisms of tumor escape in mice undergoing immunotherapy. *Cancer Research* **46**: 676–683.

Negrier S, Escudier B, Lasset C et al. (1998) Recombinant human interleukin-2, recombinant human interferon alfa-2a, or both in metastatic renal-cell carcinoma. Groupe Français d'Immunotherapie. *New England Journal of Medicine* **338**: 1272–1278.

Pizzocaro G (1986) In: de Kernion JB, Pavone Macaluso M (eds), *Tumours of the Kidney. International Perspectives in Urology.* Baltimore, MD: Williams & Wilkins.

Pizzocaro G, Piva L, Colavita M et al. (2001) Interferon adjuvant to radical nephrectomy in Robson stages II and III renal cell carcinoma: a multicentre randomised study. *Journal of Clinical Oncology* **19**: 425–431.

Porsolt F on behalf of the DELTA-P study (1992) Adjuvant therapy of renal cell cancer with interferon alpha-2a. *Proceedings of the American Society of Clinical Oncology* **11**: 202.

Rafla S, Parikh K (1984) The role of adjuvant radiotherapy in the management of renal cell cancer. In: Javadpour N (ed.), *Cancer of the Kidney.* New York: Thième-Stratton.

Selli C, Hinshaw WM, Woodard BH, Paulson DF (1983) Stratification of risk factors in renal cell carcinoma. *Cancer* **52**: 899–903.

Skinner DG, Colvin RB, Vermillion CD, Pfister RC, Leadbetter WF (1971) Diagnosis and management of renal cell carcinoma. A clinical and pathologic study of 309 cases. *Cancer* **28**: 1165–1177.

Stein M, Kuten A, Halpern J, Coachman NM, Cohen Y, Robinson E (1992) The value of postoperative irradiation in renal cell cancer. *Radiotherapy and Oncology* **24**: 41–44.

Trump DL, Elson P, Propert J and the Eastern Cooperative Group (1996) Randomised, controlled trial of adjuvant therapy with lymphoblastoid interferon in resected, high risk renal cell cancer. *Proceedings of the American Society of Clinical Oncology.*

van der Werf-Messing B, van der Heul RO, Ledchoer RCH (1978) Renal cell carcinoma trial. *Cancer Clinical Trials* **1**: 13–21.

Van Poppel H, Vandendriessche H et al. (1997) Microscopic vascular invasion is the most relevant prognosticator after radical nephrectomy for clinically non-metastatic renal cell carcinoma. *Journal of Urology* **158**: 45–49.

Vugrin D (1987) Systemic therapy of metastatic renal cell carcinoma. *Seminars in Nephrology* **7**: 152–162.

Yagoda A, Bander WH (1989) Failure of cytotoxic chemotherapy and the emerging role of monoclonal antibodies for renal cancer. *Urology International* **44**: 338–345.

Chapter 11

New approaches to immunotherapy for renal cell carcinoma

Hardev S Pandha, Agnieszka Michael and Theodora Foukaneli

The incidence of renal cell carcinoma (RCC) is rising by 2–4% per year according to recent statistics. Less than 10% of patients with stage IV disease survive 5 years, their median survival being between 7 and 11 months. To date, biological therapies have shown useful anti-cancer activity in a minority of patients; the use of chemotherapy has been limited to a combined approach with immunotherapy (biochemotherapy) and radiotherapy is essentially reserved for symptom relief, such as painful bone metastases. However, recent insights into molecular aspects of RCC and the interaction of this malignancy with the immune system have led to new treatment approaches. In this chapter, we discuss three new strategies currently under evaluation for the treatment of metastatic RCC, all of which have the common theme of immunomodulation. This is achieved by the use of specialised antigen-presenting cells called dendritic cells (DCs), the use of immunomodulating drugs such as thalidomide or by a wholly more aggressive approach using stem-cell transplantation and exploiting the powerful anti-tumour effects of graft-versus-host reactions.

Immunological aspects of renal cell carcinoma

A number of clinical observations have suggested that the immune system may be important in the behaviour of RCC *in situ*. Up to 40% of patients with RCC suffer from a variety of paraneoplastic syndromes, including fever, cachexia, hypercalcaemia, neuropathy and polycythaemia. The variable natural history of metastatic RCC, which may include prolonged disease stabilisation or spontaneous regression, raises the suspicion that the immune system may play a role in controlling this disease. Spontaneous regression has been reported in 6–7% of the placebo-treated patients enrolled in phase III trials and patients prospectively followed without treatment (Oliver et al. 1989; Young 1998). In rare instances, spontaneous regression of metastatic lesions after nephrectomy and after inflammatory or infectious events has also been reported (Young 1998). Further evidence of immune system involvement comes from the observation of dendritic cells and T cells called tumour-infiltrating lymphocytes (TILs) by immunohistochemistry, by direct cloning of TILs extracted from tumours and by in vitro stimulation of patient T-cell lines with autologous tumour cells (Finke et al. 1992). Polymerase chain reaction (PCR)-based detection methods have frequently confirmed the presence of clonal antigen-specific T cells within tumour tissue and in draining lymph nodes (Caignard et al. 1996). These T-cell clones, if extracted and expanded in culture, are capable of inducing lysis of autologous RCC in vitro (Brouwenstijn et al. 1996). TIL-based cellular therapy for RCC was successful in early clinical trials, but limited by toxicity and cost as each treatment had to be patient specific (Bukowski et al. 1991).

In most individuals with RCC, the native T-cell immune response to their disease is insufficient to control tumour progression. There is evidence that both the host immune system and tumour cells contribute to the ability of RCC to evade the immune response. The majority of TILs cloned from RCC patients are non-cytolytic CD4+ T-helper cells. When activated, these CD4+ cells are unable to secrete sufficient amounts of interleukin-2 (IL2) or interferon-γ (IFNγ) (Schoof et al. 1993). Furthermore, a number of intracellular signalling pathways involve NFκB and specific tyrosine kinases, which may be altered in T cells from RCC patients, ultimately reducing their survival. Alternatively, RCC may contribute to their own survival by producing inhibitory cytokines such as IL10, prostaglandin E2 and tumour necrosis factor-α (TNFα). Furthermore, RCC cells selectively lose expression of HLA class I alleles, enabling them to evade recognition by CD8 T cells (Luboldt et al. 1996).

The existence of antigens in association with a particular tumour that can be recognised by the immune system is critical for the generation of immune response against that tumour. Such antigens may be expressed on the cell surface and are capable of being recognised by antibodies, or may be intracellular, which can be presented by class I molecules of the major histocompatibility complex (MHC) to T cells. These antigens may be tumour specific such as viral antigens or a unique product of a mutated oncogene. Alternatively, they may be tumour associated, being expressed at abnormally high levels or at an inappropriate time (e.g. fetal antigens expressed during adulthood) (Coulie 1996). One of the key limitations in the development of specific immunotherapy for RCC has been the lack of tumour antigens specific to RCC for selective targeting. This is not surprising in view of the paucity of RCC cell lines available for in vitro study and the difficulties in raising new RCC cell lines without viral modification. However, there has been recent progress in attempts to identify new antigens or markers associated with RCC, in the hope that they may be exploited for targeted immunotherapy. None of the factors shown in Table 11.1 is specific for RCC. Some of these markers have already been evaluated in studies for their prognostic value, but do not appear to be more useful than the most robust indicators of prognosis, namely tumour stage and tumour grade. Nevertheless, and more importantly, of the new tumour antigens described, some have been found to contain specific peptide sequences (epitopes) capable, by presentation by MHC class I molecules, of being recognised by the T-cell receptor, thereby activating T cells to produce a cascade of cytolytic cytokines.

Table 11.1 Markers associated with renal cell carcinoma (RCC)

Marker	Association with RCC (%)	Other tissue in which expression may be observed
G250	85	Gut mucosa
CD44	48	Breast and colorectal carcinoma
HER-2/neu	45	Foetal heart, breast, colon, pancreas, ovarian cancers
PRAME	40	Melanoma, leukaemia, myeloma
RAGE-1	21	Retina, colorectal cancer

The presence and peptide sequence of these 'tumour rejection antigens' have been confirmed by eluting the peptides from tumour MHC class I molecule complexes and analysis by mass spectrometry. These peptide sequences can be made synthetically, or tumour cells can be modified to express them at the cell surface by gene transfer technology (by transferring the DNA sequence encoding the peptides). Immunisation with synthetic peptides, modified tumour cells or tumour lysates expressing these peptides have all resulted in useful T-cell responses. However, despite these important advances, it must be emphasised that most cancer vaccines have been based on using whole tumour cells, tumour lysates or tumour RNA, which putatively have a wide repertoire of antigens containing T-cell epitopes which may not have necessarily been identified.

Dendritic cell therapy

Dendritic cells (DCs) are the most powerful antigen-presenting cells (APCs) known (Banchereau and Steinman 1998). They are bone marrow-derived cells that normally reside in a number of tissues. They possess the specialised armamentarium for the modulation of innate and humoral immune responses, and the processing and presenting of antigens as peptide fragments to T cells. In this way, antigen-specific cytotoxic T cells (CTLs) are primed against a variety of micro-organisms as well as tumour cells. The isolation, identification and culture of DCs from bone marrow-derived precursors and monocytes have led to the development of a new field in immunotherapy (Figures 11.1 and 11.2).

Although DCs are terminally differentiated APCs, the specific properties of DCs that enable them to be used for cancer therapy are directly related to their degree of maturation. Immature DCs are characterised by high efficiency of antigen capture and processing and, as they mature, this ability is replaced by enhanced co-stimulatory function, migration to regional lymphoid tissue and activation of T cells. DCs modified by coating or 'pulsing' with peptide antigens or tumour lysate have been shown to elicit tumour-specific CTLs in vitro, and induce therapeutic responses in animal models and human studies. Responses to DC therapy have resulted in durable memory T-cell responses and regression of established disease.

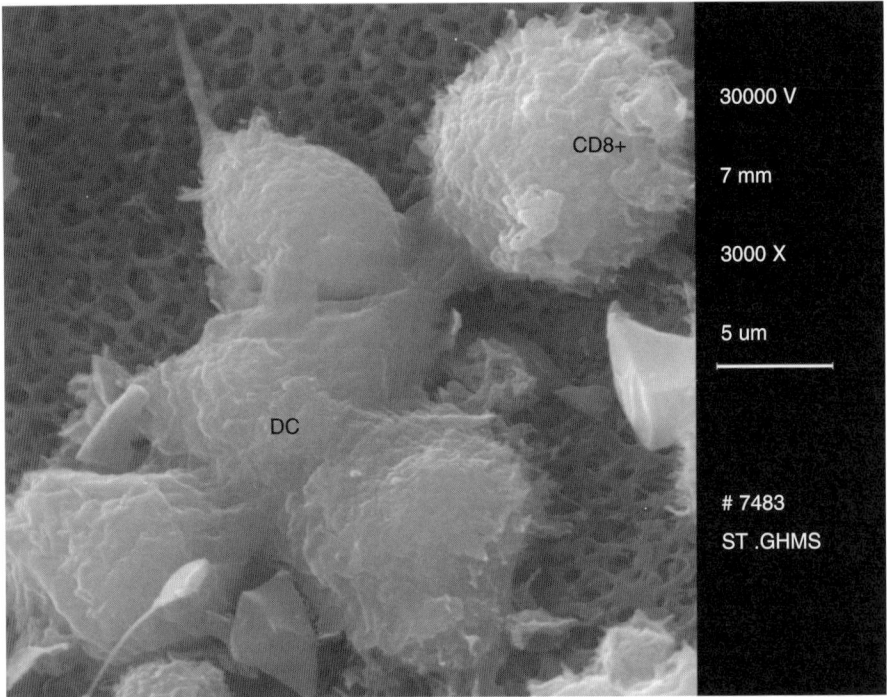

Figure 11.1 Scanning electron micrograph of a human dendritic cell (DC) interacting with a CD8+ T cell. (Reproduced by kind permission of Mr Justin John, St George's Hospital Medical School.)

The anti-tumour efficacy of DC-based therapeutic vaccines in animal models has led to a number of human trials involving sequential injections of manipulated or genetically modified cells. The marked immunogenicity of DCs has been confirmed in studies in healthy volunteers. Mature DCs pulsed with tetanus toxoid (TT), keyhole limpet haemocyanin (KLH) or influenza matrix protein (MP) peptide delivered subcutaneously, primed HLA-A2-positive individuals to KLH, and boosted underlying TT and MP responses (Dhodapkar et al. 1999). The cellular and humoral immune responses to pulsed DCs peaked 1–3 months after injection and declined by 6–9 months. Importantly, T-cell memory from the first injection was maintained because individuals re-injected with further DCs pulsed with MP also demonstrated greater, more rapid and higher MP-specific CD8+ T-cell responses (Dhodapkar et al. 2000).

Several studies have been published using DC-based immunotherapy, mostly in cancer patients with RCC, melanoma, myeloma, lymphoma or prostate cancer (Hsu et al. 1996; Nestle et al. 1998; Lim and Bailey-Wood 1999; Murphy et al. 1999; Kugler et al. 2000). Evidence of clinical improvement (e.g. regression of metastases) and enhanced T-cell immunity (antigen-specific proliferatory responses and delayed

(a)

Immature DC   Intermediate DC   Mature DC

CD34+ progenitors
bone marrow

IL-4
GM-CSF

CD14+ monocytes

CD1a+
MHC class I ^{low}
B7.1 and B7.2 ^{low}
ICAM-1 ^{low}
Macropinocytosis++

CD1a+
MHC class II ^{high}
B7.1 and B7.2 ^{high}
ICAM-1 ^{high}
Macropinocytosis–

(b)

B7.1   CD28

DC

MHC
class 1   T-cell receptor

T-cell

Proliferation
Differentation
Cytokine release,
i.e. effector function

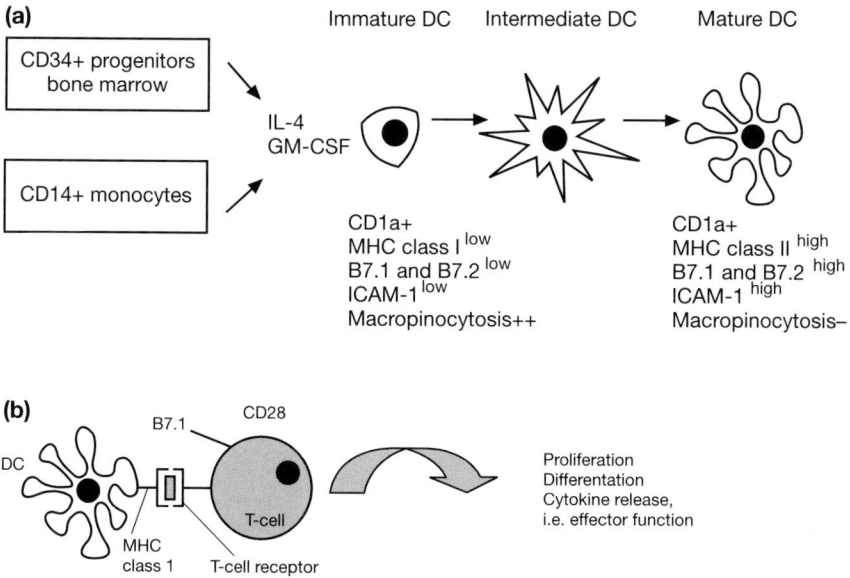

Figure 11.2 (a) Dendritic cells (DCs) may be cultured from CD34+ progenitor cells or CD14+ monocytes using specific cytokines (interleukin-4 [IL4] and granulocyte–macrophage colony-stimulating factor [GM-CSF]). Immature DCs have physiological properties (such as phagocytosis or macropinocytosis) that favour the uptake of tumour or viral antigen. Mature DCs are able to activate T-cell responses more effectively than immature cells, but are less able to take up exogenous antigen.
(b) Interaction of a DC expressing a tumour antigen on its surface (by an MHC class I molecule) with a CD8+ T cell. In order for the T cell to become activated and release cytokines to recruit further CD8+ T cells, a co-stimulatory interaction between B7.1 and CD28 is mandatory.
ICAM, intercellular adhesion molecule; MHC, major histocompatibility complex.

hypersensitivity reactions) were obtained, in some cases even in late-stage disease. As a result of differences in protocol design, effects of concurrent treatment, DC source, routes of administration, frequency of immunisation and a general lack of accepted (immunological) markers of response, the results of different DC strategies are difficult to compare. A recent study reported anti-tumour reponses from a DC vaccine comprising autologous (self) RCC cells fused with allogeneic (foreign) DCs. This approach has been shown to extremely promising in murine studies, using murine DCs and human breast cancer cell hybrids (Gong et al. 1997). Although some of the experimental details were not substantiated and the study results withdrawn, clear tumour regressions were seen (Kugler et al. 2000). It is possible that clinical improvements may have simply reflected response to autologous tumour similar to that observed in cellular immunisation in other cancers.

One of the main limitations for DC immunotherapy has been the labour cost of producing clinical grade vaccines. Patients have had to undergo repeated venesections and the quality control of consecutive vaccines cannot be guaranteed. In our own ongoing clinical DC study at St George's Hospital Medical School, we have developed a method of culturing DCs from a single large venesection, pulsing the DCs with RCC lysate and then cryopreserving aliquots of modified DCs as vaccines. In this way individual vaccine aliquots may be thawed and fully tested for phenotype, function and microbial safety before immunising the patient. Patients then receive identical vaccines at predetermined times. So far six RCC patients have received between six and ten vaccines at 2- to 4-week intervals. Data from this study should be available in early 2003.

The source, nature and method of antigen loading on dendritic cells may ultimately influence the efficacy of a DC vaccine. Microarray technology may give us a new spectrum of antigens to target in RCC. As indicated earlier, tumour antigens of many different cell constituents have already been tested in humans, including peptides, proteins, tumour lysates and tumour–DC fusions (Fong and Engleman 2000). Immunogenicity to any of these components may be improved by the development of modified high affinity peptides and inclusion of CD4-helper epitopes in the choice of antigens for vaccines (Overwijk et al. 1998). Antigens that provide multiple epitopes for both CD4+ and CD8+ T cells (cell lysates, apoptopic cells, exosomes, heat shock proteins, tumour–DC fusions, replicating and non-replicating viral vectors, and DNA- and RNA-encoding known tumour virus antigens) (Scrody et al. 2000) and antigens that simultaneously mature DCs (DNA-containing methylated CpG motifs, heat shock proteins and necrotic tumour lysates) could provide a distinct advantage over simple peptide epitopes. The use of subtractive hybridisation strategies may permit the amplification of tumour-specific RNA (Gilboa 1999). Finally, supplementing DCs with cytokines associated with T-helper-1 immunity, such as IL12, may also be important.

However, fundamental issues have still to be resolved with respect to DC vaccines. These include optimal DC dose, route of administration, frequency of immunisation and the choice of adjuvant (molecules such as Bacille Calmette–Guérin [BCG] co-administered with vaccines to boost the immune response). Once basic immunisation schedules have been established, strategies aimed at increasing DC survival and numbers in vivo may be important to prolong the period of antigenic stimulation while minimising the production costs and time. Two members of the TNF super family, CD40 ligand and TRANCE, enhance DC survival and DC immunogenicity in vitro and in vivo (Banchereau et al. 2000). The administration of the cytokine Flt-3 ligand enhances circulating dendritic cells by 50-fold, and exerts anti-tumour responses and even reverses tolerance to at least protein antigens.

A remarkable feature of all the DC vaccine studies to date has been the lack of significant acute or long-term toxicity related to DC injections. The development of slight fever or myalgia, the main toxicity reported, may be related to the use of fetal calf serum in the DC culture. Autoimmunity (as vitiligo) has been described in a melanoma DC study, where effective tumour immunity was observed, presumably as a result of cross-priming of tumour antigens (Banchereau et al. 2001). This is a timely reminder of potential toxicity when targeting antigens that are shared by tumour cells and normal cells. Despite vigorous in vitro manipulation and modification, there has been no report of a dendritic cell malignancy to date.

Immunomodulatory drugs: thalidomide and its analogues

Thalidomide (α-N-phthalidomidoglutarimide) is a synthetic derivative of glutamic acid and was first synthesised in the 1950s. Its teratogenicity and neurotoxicity led to its removal from the market as a treatment for pregnancy-associated nausea. Thalidomide has been in almost continuous but highly selective use since then. These applications include erythema nodosum leprosum (Sheskin 1965), as an immunosuppressive agent for the treatment of chronic graft-versus-host disease (Vogelsang et al. 1992) and a number of inflammatory conditions, including rheumatoid arthritis, Behçet's disease and Crohn's disease (Schuler and Ehninger 1995; Wettstein and Meagher 1997; Hamuryudan et al. 1998). More recently, thalidomide has been shown to be effective in the treatment of oral ulceration and cachexia associated with HIV infection and AIDS-related Kaposi's sarcoma (Sharpstone et al. 1995; Fife et al. 1998).

Thalidomide has been shown to have both anti-inflammatory and immuno-modulatory activity. It is able to inhibit the synthesis of TNFα, a pro-inflammatory cytokine produced by activated human monocytes (Sampaio et al. 1991). TNFα is a key regulator of other pro-inflammatory cytokines and leukocyte adhesion molecules (Eigler et al. 2001). The presence of thalidomide alters the cytokine environment by the inhibition of specific cytokines such as interleukin-12 (IL12) and the increase in other cytokines such as IL4. Thalidomide may also be able to activate T cells in the absence of co-stimulatory signals. Other effects include oxidative DNA damage by generation of hydroxyl free radicals (Sauer et al. 2000) and downregulation of cell-surface adhesion receptors (Thiel et al. 2000). Tumour growth has been shown to be dependent on angiogenesis (or the formation of new blood vessels), which correlates with the likelihood of developing metastases and overall prognosis in patients (Folkman 1995). TNFα is involved in the upregulation of endothelial integrin expression, a process important in the formation of new blood vessels (Ruegg et al. 1998). Thalidomide has been shown to exert anti-angiogenic activity in murine models, which may explain the pattern of limb defects in the developing fetus that brought it to notoriety in the 1960s (Ching et al. 1995). The toxicity of thalidomide includes peripheral neuropathy, constipation, mucositis and somnolence. It has been suggested that, as thalidomide is currently used as a racemic mixture, the administration of a single enantiomer rather than the racemic mixture may improve the side-effect profile.

Clinical trials of thalidomide in RCC

Thalidomide has been evaluated in a number of solid malignancies and in refractory multiple myeloma (Singhal et al. 1999; Eisen et al. 2000). An initial study of low-dose (100 mg) thalidomide in a variety of solid tumours indicated some useful activity (objective responses and stable disease) in RCC, consistent with unpublished reports from other centres (Eisen et al. 2000). A follow-up study involved 25 patients treated with up to 600 mg thalidomide daily. Two patients showed partial response, seven had stable disease for over 6 months and five stable disease for between 3 and 6 months. There was no survival advantage. The most common toxicities (lethargy, constipation and neuropathy) were of sufficient clinical significance to justify a lower well-tolerated dose (400 mg) of this drug (Stebbing et al. 2001).

There have been efforts to harness the beneficial effects of thalidomide by the development of a number of thalidomide analogues. These new agents can be usefully divided into two groups based on their proposed mechanism of action. Both are potent inhibitors of TNFα. They have been termed 'selective cytokine inhibitory drugs' (SelCIDs) and 'immunomodulatory drugs' (ImiDs). All the SelCID analogues are phosphodiesterase type IV inhibitors; inhibition of this enzyme correlates well with TNFα inhibition after stimulation of a specific monocytic cell line. The ImiD analogues have no effect of phosphodiesterase type 4 and act through an as yet unknown mechanism (Horowitz et al. 1990; Corral et al. 1998; Muller et al. 1996, 1999). Both types of analogue are currently being evaluated in the treatment of multiple myeloma, renal cancer, melanoma and pancreatic carcinoma.

Immune modulation using stem-cell transplantation

Allogeneic bone marrow transplantation was developed as a method to replace diseased marrow in patients with primary disorders of the bone marrow. At the same time, it enabled the escalation of chemotherapy and radiotherapy doses in patients with malignant disease. Although the ultimate value of haematopoietic stem-cell transplantation has yet to be established, there is little doubt that many patients would not survive without this treatment. Conditions for which allogeneic bone marrow transplantation may be undertaken include malignant haematological disorders (leukaemia, lymphoma multiple myeloma), congenital immunodeficiency syndromes and disorders characterised by defective haematopoiesis. In the past, stem cells were obtained from the bone marrow, but more recently peripheral blood and placental blood have proved to be effective sources of these cells. During the bone marrow transplantation, after the appropriate conditioning (cytotoxic therapy or radiotherapy) and re-infusion of the stem cells, the donor-derived stem cells re-populate the damaged or ablated bone marrow of the recipient. Graft rejection and graft-versus-host disease (GVHD) are two of the major complications of transplantation. GVHD disease is the term describing an immunological attack by the donor lymphocytes that recognise host tissues as foreign. Clinical and experimental data have established that the pathogenesis of GVHD requires the transfer of donor-derived T lymphocytes with the stem cells. In several haematological disorders, in particular in chronic myelogenous leukaemia, the development of GVHD is associated with a lower incidence of disease relapse (Horowitz et al. 1990).

It is also known that T-cell-depleted bone marrow or bone marrow derived from identical twins is associated with an increased relapse rate (Weiden et al. 1979). These findings are suggestive of a separate graft-versus-tumour (GVT) mechanism that accompanies GVHD. Donor T cells play an important role for the development of both GVHD and GVT (Eibl et al. 1996; Verdonck et al. 1996; van Besien et al. 1997). For patients who relapse despite successful initial engraftment, further immune manipulation is possible using infusions of the donor's lymphocytes (DLI) to provoke GVHD and GVT (Kolb et al. 1995; Slavin et al. 1996). These patients may actually have durable remission without the additional use of chemotherapy. Interestingly, many patients have achieved a GVT (or specifically a graft versus leukaemia) response without developing GVHD, which can be explained by the presence of different antigens involved with each process. It could also result from a greater sensitivity of malignant cells than visceral tissues to a common immunological mechanism. Both CD4+ and CD8+ T cells participate in the initiation of GVHD. Other cell populations including natural killer (NK) cells and cytokines participate as mediators of tissue injury (Korngold and Sprent 1987; Sakamoto et al. 1991). A major challenge clearly is to separate the beneficial GVT from the manifestations of GVHD.

Non-myeloablative stem-cell transplantations

Transplantation-related mortality results partly from the side effects of myeloablative conditioning and partly from the GVHD and delayed recovery of cell-mediated immunity. To exploit the GVT effect in patients who could not tolerate high-dose chemotherapy, new strategies have been developed. These include: first, the use of reduced intensive preparative regimens, insufficient to destroy the recipient bone marrow permanently but sufficient to allow donor stem-cell engraftment; second, the induction of tolerance between the host and the donor immune system and prevention of the development of GVHD – in many cases the resulting peripheral leucocytes contain both donor and host cells, and are referred to as chimaeric; and, finally, optimising the donor immune recovery and the GVT effect by increasing the speed and completeness of donor immune recovery. For the last purpose donor lymphocyte infusion and short-term immunosuppression follow the transplantation. These approaches are collectively grouped under the term 'non-myeloablative stem-cell transplants' or 'mini-transplants'.

The use of lower-dose chemotherapy reduces toxicity and may improve the outcome of the patients at high risk of dying from transplantation-related causes. In combination with the GVT effect, which may alone be sufficient to cure some haematological malignancies, this has been used successfully in several series of patients with haematological malignancies, including acute or chronic leukaemia, non-Hodgkin's lymphoma, myelodysplastic syndrome or multiple myeloma (Slavin et al. 1998; Childs et al. 1999a).

Non-myeloablative allotransplantation in metastatic RCC

Metastatic RCC is resistant to cytotoxic therapies, but does respond to cytokine therapy in a minority of patients. Previous reports suggested that a GVT effect does occur in non-haematological malignancies, as seen in breast cancer. Attempts have been made to use this approach in RCC but with the improved safety of the non-myeloablative procedure. In 1999, Childs et al. (1999b) presented a case report suggesting a graft-versus-RCC effect using non-myeloablative allogeneic stem-cell transplantation. This was followed by a pilot study of 19 patients with metastatic RCC refractory to conventional cytokine and chemotherapy (Childs et al. 2000). All patients had a stem-cell donor who was an HLA identical or HLA single antigen-mismatched sibling. Patients received pre-transplantation conditioning chemotherapy comprising cyclophosphamide and fludarabine – two agents that otherwise have little or no single agent activity in this disease. Stem cells were infused into the recipient without T-cell depletion. Cyclosporin was used as GVHD prophylaxis, but was tapered down over 2 weeks in patients who had persistent host T cells. Then up to three donor lymphocyte infusions (DLIs) were administered until the entire T-cell population was donor derived; the patient developed GVHD or there was evidence of regression of the RCC. In addition, low dose of subcutaneous IFNα or IL2 was administered to stimulate an immune response in some patients who had no disease response to DLI, or who were not candidates for DLI because of GVHD. Despite these variations in post-transplantation drug therapy, a number of conclusions were drawn. Of the 19 patients evaluated, two died from transplantation causes and eight from progressive disease. There were three complete responses and seven partial responses. Regression of metastases was delayed, occurring a median of 129 days after transplantation, following the withdrawal of cyclosporin and establishment of complete donor T-cell chimaerism. This is consistent with a GVT effect (Figure 11.3).

Although the use of non-myeloablative allogeneic stem-cell transplantation for treatment of RCC is still in the preliminary stages, the result of the Childs' study results demonstrated the feasibility of the approach and highlighted the potential toxicities. The optimal preparative regimen intensity, the type of chemotherapy, and the inclusion or otherwise of radiotherapy will be made clear only by further clinical trials. As with haematological malignancies treated by mini-allogeneic transplantation, key issues such as the incidence of acute and chronic GVHD, GVHD prophylaxis and the use of DLI need to be addressed. For now, stem-cell transplantation for solid tumours remains experimental and should be carried out only in the context of a clinical trial. This will then allow us to make a careful evaluation of the potential use

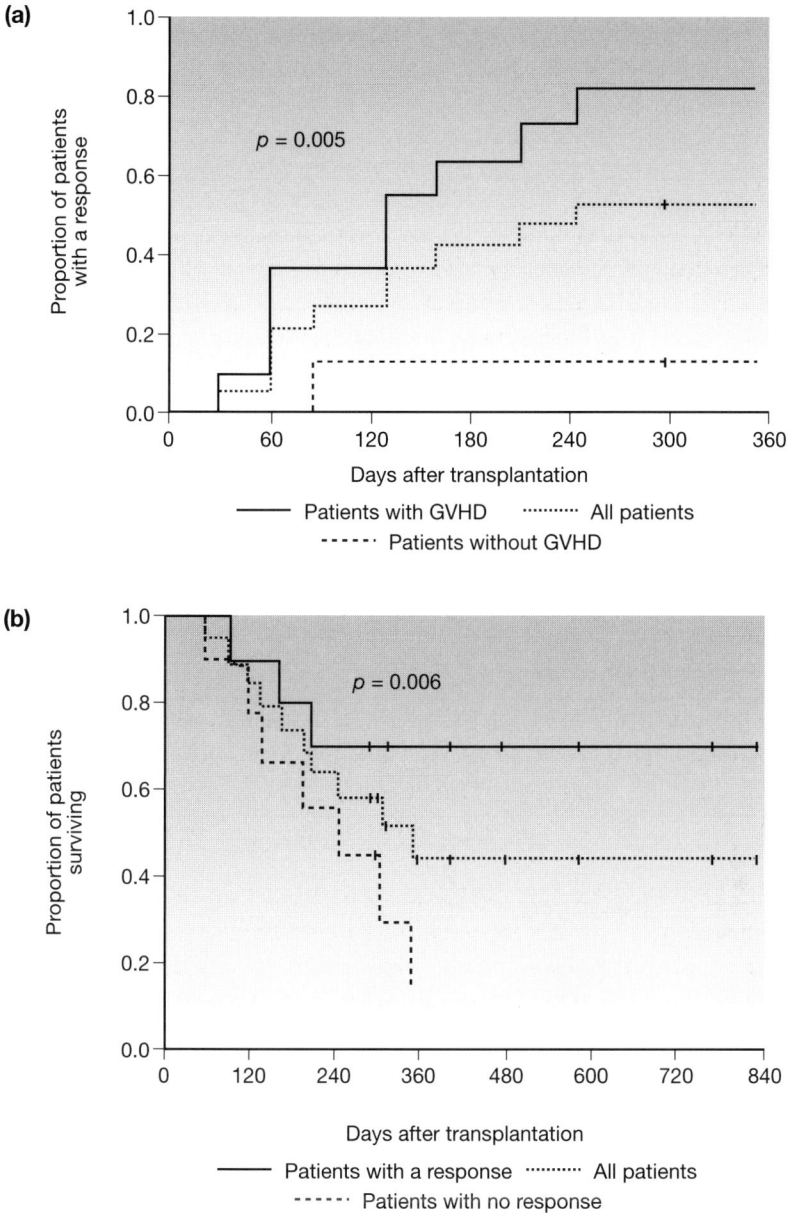

Figure 11.3 (a) The appearance of a GVHD is associated with an anti-tumour response. **(b)** An anti-tumour response is associated with an overall survival benefit. (Reproduced with permission from the *New England Journal of Medicine.*)

of mismatched and matched, unrelated donors because we expect that many RCC patients will not necessarily have suitable sibling matches for stem-cell donation.

Conclusion

Metastatic RCC, although a rare cancer, remains a difficult clinical condition to treat. Current therapies remain unsatisfactory, with limited efficacy and high toxicity. New insights into immunological aspects of RCC have resulted in new attempts at modulating the immune system for therapeutic purposes. New clinical trials include the use of modified dendritic cells, immunomodulatory drugs such as thalidomide and its analogues, as well as potentially more toxic approaches involving stem-cell transplantation. For our patients, we have great hopes that one or more of these approaches will result in durable responses and prolonged survival. It is clear that, where there is potentially life-threatening toxicity, coordinated clinical trials and careful patients selection will be vital.

References

Banchereau J, Steinman RM (1998) Dendritic cells and the control of immunity. *Nature* **392**: 245–252.

Banchereau J, Briere F, Caux C et al. (2000) Immunobiology of dendritic cells. *Annual Review of Immunology* **18**: 767–811.

Banchereau J, Palucka AK, Dhodapkar M et al. (2001) Immune and clinical responses in patients with metastatic melanoma to CD34(+) progenitor-derived dendritic cell vaccine. *Cancer Research* **61**: 6451–6458.

Brouwenstijn N, Gaugler B, Kruse KM et al. (1996) Renal-cell carcinoma-specific lysis by cytotoxic T-lymphocyte clones isolated from peripheral blood lymphocytes and tumor-infiltrating lymphocytes. *International Journal of Cancer* **68**: 177–182.

Bukowski RM, Sharfman W, Murthy S et al. (1991) Clinical results and characterization of tumor-infiltrating lymphocytes with or without recombinant interleukin 2 in human metastatic renal cell carcinoma. *Cancer Research* **51**: 4199–205.

Caignard A, Guillard M, Gaudin C, Escudier B, Triebel F, Dietrich PY (1996) In situ demonstration of renal-cell-carcinoma-specific T-cell clones. *International Journal of Cancer* **66**: 564–570.

Childs R, Clave E, Contentin N et al. (1999a) Engraftment kinetics after nonmyeloablative allogeneic peripheral blood stem cell transplantation: full donor T-cell chimerism precedes alloimmune responses. *Blood* **94**: 3234–3241.

Childs RW, Clave E, Tisdale J, Plante M, Hensel N, Barrett J (1999b) Successful treatment of metastatic renal cell carcinoma with a nonmyeloablative allogeneic peripheral-blood progenitor-cell transplant: evidence for a graft-versus-tumor effect. *Journal of Clinical Oncology* **17**: 2044–2049.

Childs R, Chernoff A, Contentin N et al. (2000) Regression of metastatic renal-cell carcinoma after nonmyeloablative allogeneic peripheral-blood stem-cell transplantation. *New England Journal of Medicine* **343**: 750–758.

Ching LM, Xu ZF, Gummer BH, Palmer BD, Joseph WR, Baguley BC (1995) Effect of thalidomide on tumour necrosis factor production and anti- tumour activity induced by 5,6-dimethylxanthenone-4-acetic acid. *British Journal of Cancer* **72**: 339–343.

Corral LG, Muller GW, Moreira AL et al. (1996) Selection of novel analogs of thalidomide with enhanced tumor necrosis factor alpha inhibitory activity. *Molecular Medicine* **2**: 506–515.

Coulie P (1996) Human tumour antigens recognised by cytolytic T lymphocytes. In: Dalgleish A, Browning M (eds), *Tumour Immunology*. Cambridge: Cambridge University Press, pp. 95–125.

Dhodapkar MV, Steinman RM, Sapp M et al. (1999) Rapid generation of broad T-cell immunity in humans after a single injection of mature dendritic cells. *Journal of Clinical Investigation* **104**: 173–180.

Dhodapkar MV, Krasovsky J, Steinman RM, Bhardwaj N (2000) Mature dendritic cells boost functionally superior CD8(+) T-cell in humans without foreign helper epitopes. *Journal of Clinical Investigation* **105**: R9–R14.

Eibl B, Schwaighofer H, Nachbaur D et al. (1996) Evidence for a graft-versus-tumor effect in a patient treated with marrow ablative chemotherapy and allogeneic bone marrow transplantation for breast cancer. *Blood* **88**: 1501–1508.

Eigler A, Loher F, Endres S (2001) Suppression of synthesis of tumor necrosis factor [in German]. *Internist (Berlin)* **42**(1): 28–34.

Eisen T, Boshoff C, Mak I et al. (2000) Continuous low dose thalidomide: a phase II study in advanced melanoma, renal cell, ovarian and breast cancer. *British Journal of Cancer* **82**: 812–817.

Fife K, Howard MR, Gracie F, Phillips RH, Bower M (1998) Activity of thalidomide in AIDS-related Kaposi's sarcoma and correlation with HHV8 titre. *International Journal of STD and AIDS* **9**: 751–755.

Finke JH, Rayman P, Edinger M et al. (1992) Characterization of a human renal cell carcinoma specific cytotoxic CD8+ T cell line. *Journal of Immunotherapy* **11**: 1–11.

Folkman J (1995) Seminars in medicine of the Beth Israel Hospital, Boston. Clinical applications of research on angiogenesis. *New England Journal of Medicine* **333**: 1757–1763.

Fong L, Engleman EG (2000) Dendritic cells in cancer immunotherapy. *Annual Review of Immunology* **18**: 245–273.

Gilboa E (1999) The makings of a tumor rejection antigen. *Immunity* **11**: 263–270.

Gong J, Chen D, Kashiwaba M, Kufe D (1997) Induction of antitumor activity by immunization with fusions of dendritic and carcinoma cells. *Nature Medicine* **3**: 558–561.

Hamuryudan V, Mat C, Saip S et al. (1998) Thalidomide in the treatment of the mucocutaneous lesions of the Behçet syndrome. A randomized, double-blind, placebo-controlled trial. *Annals of Internal Medicine* **128**: 443–450.

Horowitz MM, Gale RP, Sondel PM et al. (1990) Graft-versus-leukemia reactions after bone marrow transplantation. *Blood* **75**: 555–562.

Hsu FJ, Benike C, Fagnoni F et al. (1996) Vaccination of patients with B-cell lymphoma using autologous antigen-pulsed dendritic cells. *Nature Medicine* **2**(1): 52–58.

Kolb HJ, Schattenberg A, Goldman JM et al. (1995) Graft-versus-leukemia effect of donor lymphocyte transfusions in marrow grafted patients. European Group for Blood and Marrow Transplantation Working Party Chronic Leukemia. *Blood* **86**: 2041–2050.

Korngold R, Sprent J (1987) T cell subsets and graft-versus-host disease. *Transplantation* **44**: 335–359.

Kugler A, Stuhler G, Walden P et al. (2000) Regression of human metastatic renal cell carcinoma after vaccination with tumor cell-dendritic cell hybrids. *Nature Medicine* **6**: 332–336.

Lim SH, Bailey-Wood R (1999) Idiotypic protein-pulsed dendritic cell vaccination in multiple myeloma. *International Journal of Cancer* **83**: 215–222.

Luboldt HJ, Kubens BS, Rubben H, Grosse-Wilde H (1996) Selective loss of human leukocyte antigen class I allele expression in advanced renal cell carcinoma. *Cancer Research* **56**(4): 826–30.

Muller GW, Chen R, Huang SY et al. (1999) Amino-substituted thalidomide analogs: potent inhibitors of TNF-alpha production. *Bioorganic Medical and Chemical Letters* **9**: 1625–1630.

Muller GW, Corral LG, Shire MG et al. (1996) Structural modifications of thalidomide produce analogs with enhanced tumor necrosis factor inhibitory activity. *Journal of Medical Chemistry* **39**: 3238–3240.

Muller GW, Shire MG, Wong LM et al. (1998) Thalidomide analogs and PDE4 inhibition. *Bioorganic Medical and Chemical Letters* **8**: 2669–2674.

Murphy GP (1999) Review of phase II hormone refractory prostate cancer trials. *Urology* **54**(6A suppl): 19–21.

Nestle FO, Alijagic S, Gilliet M et al. (1998) Vaccination of melanoma patients with peptide- or tumor lysate-pulsed dendritic cells. *Nature Medicine* **4**: 328–332.

Oliver RT, Nethersell AB, Bottomley JM (1989) Unexplained spontaneous regression and alpha-interferon as treatment for metastatic renal carcinoma. *British Journal of Urology* **63**(2): 128–131.

Overwijk WW, Tsung A, Irvine KR et al. (1998) gp100/pmel 17 is a murine tumor rejection antigen: induction of 'self'- reactive, tumoricidal T cells using high-affinity, altered peptide ligand. *Journal of Experimental Medicine* **188**: 277–2.

Ruegg C, Yilmaz A, Bieler G, Bamat J, Chaubert P, Lejeune FJ (1998) Evidence for the involvement of endothelial cell integrin alphaVbeta3 in the disruption of the tumor vasculature induced by TNF and IFN-gamma. *Nature Medicine* **4**: 408–414.

Sakamoto H, Michaelson J, Jones WK et al. (1991) Lymphocytes with a CD4+ CD8- CD3- phenotype are effectors of experimental cutaneous graft-versus-host disease. *Proceedings of the National Academy of Science of the USA* **88**: 10890–10894.

Sampaio EP, Sarno EN, Galilly R, Cohn ZA, Kaplan G (1991) Thalidomide selectively inhibits tumor necrosis factor alpha production by stimulated human monocytes. *Journal of Experimental Medicine* **173**: 699–703.

Sauer H, Gunther J, Hescheler J, Wartenberg M (2000) Thalidomide inhibits angiogenesis in embryoid bodies by the generation of hydroxyl radicals. *American Journal of Pathology* **156**: 151–158.

Schoof DD, Terashima Y, Peoples GE et al. (1993) CD4+ T cell clones isolated from human renal cell carcinoma possess the functional characteristics of Th2 helper cells. *Cell Immunology* **150**: 114–123.

Schuler U, Ehninger G (1995) Thalidomide: rationale for renewed use in immunological disorders. *Drug Safety* **12**: 364–369.

Serody JS, Collins EJ, Tisch RM, Kuhns JJ, Frelinger JA (2000) T cell activity after dendritic cell vaccination is dependent on both the type of antigen and the mode of delivery. *Journal of Immunology* **164**: 4961–4967.

Sharpstone D, Rowbottom A, Nelson M, Gazzard B (1995) The treatment of microsporidial diarrhoea with thalidomide. *Aids* **9**: 658–659.

Sheskin J (1965) Further observation with thalidomide in lepra reactions. *Leprosy Review* **36**: 183–187.

Singhal S, Mehta J, Desikan R et al. (1999) Antitumor activity of thalidomide in refractory multiple myeloma. *New England Journal of Medicine* **341**: 1565–1571.

Slavin S, Naparstek E, Nagler A et al. (1996) Allogeneic cell therapy with donor peripheral blood cells and recombinant human interleukin-2 to treat leukemia relapse after allogeneic bone marrow transplantation. *Blood* **87**: 2195–2204.

Slavin S, Nagler A, Naparstek E et al. (1998) Nonmyeloablative stem cell transplantation and cell therapy as an alternative to conventional bone marrow transplantation with lethal cytoreduction for the treatment of malignant and nonmalignant hematologic diseases. *Blood* **91**: 756–763.

Stebbing J, Benson C, Eisen T et al. (2001) The treatment of advanced renal cell cancer with high-dose oral thalidomide. *British Journal of Cancer* **85**: 953–958.

Thiel R, Kastner U, Neubert R (2000) Expression of adhesion receptors on rat limb bud cells and results of treatment with a thalidomide derivative. *Life Sciences* **66**: 133–141.

van Besien KW, de Lima M, Giralt SA et al. (1997) Management of lymphoma recurrence after allogeneic transplantation: the relevance of graft-versus-lymphoma effect. *Bone Marrow Transplantation* **19**: 977–982.

Verdonck LF, Lokhorst HM, Dekker AW, Nieuwenhuis HK, Petersen EJ (1996) Graft-versus-myeloma effect in two cases. *The Lancet* **347**: 800–801.

Vogelsang GB, Farmer ER, Hess AD et al. (1992) Thalidomide for the treatment of chronic graft-versus-host disease. *New England Journal of Medicine* **326**: 1055–1058.

Weiden PL, Flournoy N, Thomas ED et al. (1979) Antileukemic effect of graft-versus-host disease in human recipients of allogeneic-marrow grafts. *New England Journal of Medicine* **300**: 1068–1073.

Wettstein AR, Meagher AP (1997) Thalidomide in Crohn's disease. *The Lancet* **350**: 1445–1446.

Young R (1998) Metastatic renal cell carcinoma: what causes occasional dramatic regresssions? *New England Journal of Medicine* **338**: 1305–1306.

Chapter 12

An overview of prognostic factors of direct relevance to disease management

Nicholas D James and David C Wilson

Introduction

As with most cancers, prognosis depends on a variety of factors, both host- and tumour-derived. Renal cancer has an extremely variable prognosis and stage alone does not adequately describe the full range of prognostic possibilities. As there is growing evidence that certain treatments for relapsed or metastatic disease may improve survival, it has become increasingly important to assess prognosis accurately to allow effective case selection. This is particularly true as palliative options now include nephrectomy (improvement in median survival of around 50%) (Flanigan et al. 2000) and immunotherapy with interferon (improvement in median survival of around 28%) (Anonymous 1999). Clearly for patients to derive worthwhile benefit, it is essential that they have a reasonable estimated survival in the first place. Several factors need to be considered in assessing prognosis. The principal elements are: (1) pathology; (2) performance status; (3) stage. Choice of treatment is also an important factor, with several studies identifying factors such as radiotherapy dose (Onufrey & Mohiuddin 1985; DiBiase et al. 1997), and immunotherapy versus chemotherapy (Motzer et al. 2000) as having a bearing on outcome.

Pathology

Renal cell carcinomas arise from the proximal renal tubular epithelium and tend to be spherical with an average diameter of around 7 cm, though they can reach enormous sizes. There is often a pseudocapsule formed by a rim of compressed kidney with haemorrhage, and necrosis with sclerosis and fibrosis. Calcification and single or multiple fluid-filled cysts may also be seen. Tumours are usually solitary, except in familial forms of the disease. Several cellular variants have been described: clear cell, granular cell and spindle or sarcomatoid cell, and frequently tumours contain more than one type of cell morphology. Between 1% and 6% of renal tumours are sarcomatoid which are associated with a poorer prognosis (Ro et al. 1987; Selal et al. 1987). Tumours can also be graded according to the Fuhrman system (Fuhrman et al. 1982), which utilises four nuclear grades (1–4) defined in order of increasing nuclear size, irregularity and nucleolar prominence. Figure 12.1b shows survival according to nuclear grade (Zisman et al. 2001).

As predicted from experience with other malignancies such as breast carcinoma, prognosis in renal cell carcinoma is determined by the particular biology of a tumour. Several molecular markers have been identified which reflect tumour biology, particularly the rate of cell proliferation, and thus, reflect prognosis. A high proliferation index, as reflected by expression of PCNA (proliferating cell nuclear antigen) MIB-1 or Ki-67 is associated with a poorer prognosis (Lipponen et al. 1994; Pappadopoulos et al. 1996; Tannapfel et al. 1996; de Riese et al. 1993). Diploidy has also been shown to be associated with a longer disease-free interval (Di Silverio et al. 2000). Such markers may have a role to play in the selection of the suitability of palliative treatment.

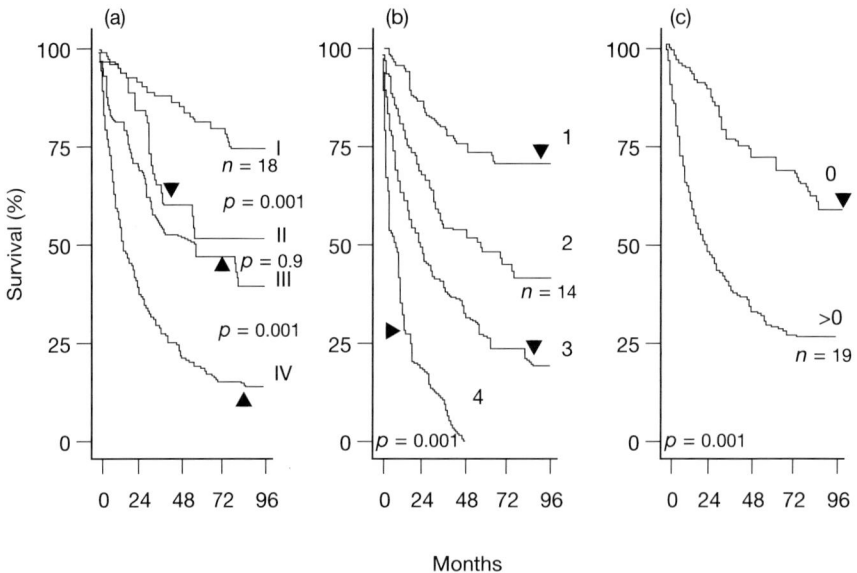

Figure 12.1 Survival by stage, Fuhrman grade and performance status.

Stage

The most widely used staging systems are the Robson system and the 1997 Consensus TNM (tumour–node–metastasis) system (see Table 12.1). Prognosis by stage is given in Figure 12.1a using the stage grouping system. As would be expected there are wide variations in survival by stage with around 75% of stage I patients alive after 7 years compared with 20% of stage IV. However, even for the worst prognostic group, there are significant numbers of long-term survivors.

Table 12.1 TNM Staging

T stage	
T1	Tumour < 7 cm
T2	Tumour > 7 cm
T3	Involvement of major veins,
T3a	Invasion of adrenal or perinephric tissue but not beyond Gerota's fascia
T3b	Invasion of renal vein or IVC below diaphragm
T3c	Invasion of renal vein above diaphragm
T4	Invasion beyond Gerota's fascia
N stage	
N0	No node involvement
N1	Single regional node
N2	> 1 Regional node involved
M stage	
M0	No metastases
M1	Distant metastases
TNM Stage Grouping	
Stage I	T1 N0 M0
Stage II	T2 N0 M0
Stage III	T1 N1 M0
	T2 N1 M0
	T3 N0/1 M0
Stage IV	T4 N0/1 M0
	Any T N2 M0
	Any T Any N M1

Performance status

The presence of systemic symptoms has a substantial effect on survival independent of stage as illustrated in Figure 12.1c, which splits the patients into ECOG PS 0 and 1 or greater. This is therefore an important factor in deciding on treatment, as it is an easily assessed variable.

A recent publication attempted to synthesise the above three variables into a unified staging system which potentially represents a useful step forward in the care of patients with renal cell carcinoma. By using a Cox regression model, patients were split into five prognostic categories. Survival of these groups is shown in Figure 12.2 and Table 12.2.

In metastatic disease, a poor performance status is consistently a factor found by multivariate analysis to have an adverse effect on prognosis (Motzer et al. 1999; Elson et al. 1988). Performance status is similarly found to be a predictive factor in response to palliative treatments such as radiotherapy (DiBiase et al. 1997).

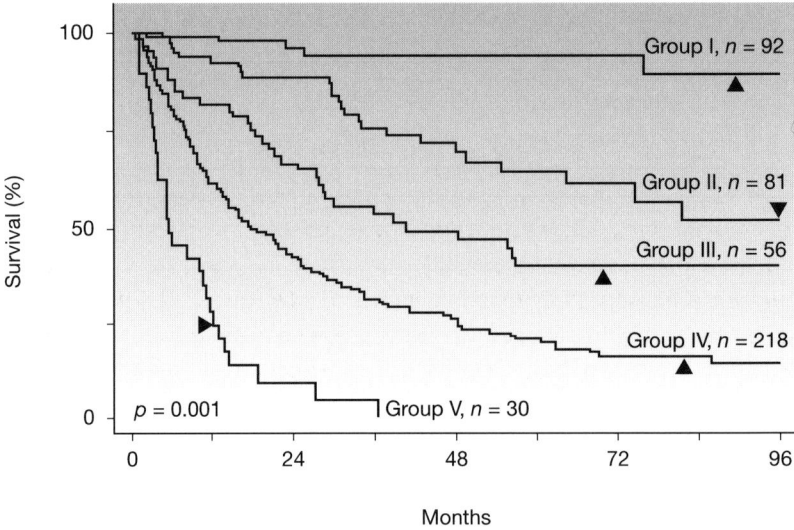

Figure 12.2 Survival by UCLA Integrated Staging System (UISS) Categories.

Table 12.2 UISS Staging system

UISS	1997 TNM stage	Furman's grade	ECOG	2-Year survival %	2-Year survival SE	5-Year survival %	5-Year survival SE
I	I	1, 2	0	96	2.5	94	2.5
II	I	1, 2	1 or more	89	3.8	67	6.4
	I	3, 4	Any				
	II	Any	Any				
	III	Any	0				
	III	1	1 or more				
III	III	2–4	1 or more	66	6.5	39	2.8
	IV	1, 2	0				
IV	IV	3, 4	0	42	3.5	23	3.1
		1–3	1 or more				
V	IV	4	1 or more	9	6.2	0	4.0

TNM, tumour–node–metastasis.

Prognosis by treatment given

Several studies have looked at the effect of treatment on survival (Motzer et al. 1999, 2000; Elson et al. 1988). Nephrectomy is consistently shown to improve prognosis (Motzer et al. 1999), including two randomised trials presented at ASCO in 2000 (Flanigan et al. 2000). In some of these studies, patients receiving chemotherapy appear to have had a worse survival than those receiving immunotherapy (Motzer et al. 2000), although these are not randomised studies. None the less, there is little evidence to support the use of currently available chemotherapy regimens and thus chemotherapy should only be given in the setting of a clinical trial.

Dose of radiotherapy versus palliative effect

Renal cell carcinoma has often been considered to be a radio-resistant tumour. However, several studies have shown that high palliative response rates may be achieved by using radiation in patients with stage IV, metastatic disease dose (Halperin and Harisiadis 1983; Onufrey et al. 1985; DiBiase et al. 1997). A recent study at the authors' institution has shown a response rate of around 75% (complete and partial response) for palliative radiotherapy to various sites (Wilson et al. 2003).

The relation between the dose of radiotherapy and palliative response has been explored in several studies to ascertain if a higher dose of radiation predicts for a better or longer response. These are summarised in Table 12.3. Briefly, two studies have suggested that higher dose predicts for a greater response rate, and two studies including one recent study at the authors institution has shown no relation between dose and either response rate or duration of response.

Table 12.3 Palliative radiotherapy

Author	n	Sites	RR (%)	Comment
Onufrey et al. (1985)	125	bone, brain, soft tissue, lung	65%	Dose–response observed. Higher response for TDF > 70 (65%) vs 25% for TDF < 70.
DiBiase et al. (1997)	150	bone, brain, soft tissue, lung	86%	Dose–response observed. Higher complete palliative response for BED > 50 (59%) vs 39% for BED< 50 ($p = 0.001$)
Halperin and Harisiadis (1983)	60	bone, brain, soft (77% tissue, lung, bone)	64%	No dose–response observed
Wilson et al. (2003)	139	bone, brain, soft tissue, lung	75%	No dose–response observed

TDF, tumour dose fractionation; BED, biological effective dose, calculated by using an alpha/beta ratio = 10.

Other means of palliation

Patients with metastatic renal cell carcinoma have a poor prognosis and will receive a range of treatments such as analgesics as part of the management of the condition. One specific tool that is widely used, both for the primary and for secondary lesions, is therapeutic embolisation. At present, there is no evidence that this has an impact on survival however (Lin et al. 2003; Munro et al. 2001; Manke et al. 2001). For patients with spinal cord compression, however, there is evidence that decompressive surgery plus stabilisation not only improves neurological outcome but also improves survival (Patchell et al. 2003). As patients with renal cell carcinoma frequently have low numbers of often very destructive lesions and relatively long survivals, they may be paticularly suited to this approach.

Conclusion

Prognosis of renal cancer is affected both by disease and treatment-related factors. A careful appraisal of the likely prognosis with different treatment options should be made as well as the likely toxicity associated with these options, which may be substantial for some of the surgical approaches listed above.

References

Anonymous (1999). Interferon-alpha and survival in metastatic renal carcinoma: early results of a randomised controlled trial. Medical Research Council Renal Cancer Collaborators. *Lancet* **353**: 14–17.

de Riese WT, Crabtree WN, Allhoff EP et al. (1993) Prognostic significance of Ki-67 immunostaining in nonmetastatic renal cell carcinoma. *Journal of Clinical Oncology* **11**: 1804–1808.

DiBiase SJ, Valicenti RK, Schultz D, Xie Y, Gomella LG, Corn BW (1997) Palliative irradiation for focally symptomatic metastatic renal cell carcinoma: support for dose escalation based on a biological model. *Journal of Urology* **158**: 746–749.

Di Silverio F, Casale P, Colella D, Andrea L, Seccareccia F, Sciarra A (2000) Independent value of tumor size and DNA ploidy for the prediction of disease progression in patients with organ-confined renal cell carcinoma. *Cancer* **88**: 835–843.

Elson PJ, Witte RS, Trump DL (1988) Prognostic factors for survival in patients with recurrent or metastatic renal cell carcinoma. *Cancer Research* **48**: 7310–7313.

Flanigan RC, Blumenstein BA, Salmon S, Crawford ED (2000) Cytoreduction nephrectomy in metastatic renal cancer: the results of Southwest Oncology Group Trial 8949. *Proceedings of the American Society of Clinical Oncology* **200**: 1393 (abstract).

Fuhrman SA, Lasky LC, Limas C (1982) Prognostic significance of morphologic parameters in renal cell carcinoma. *American Journal of Surgical Pathology* **6**: 655–663.

Halperin EC, Harisiadis L (1983) The role of radiation therapy in the management of metastatic renal cell carcinoma. *Cancer* **51**: 614–617.

Lin PH, Terramani TT, Bush RL, Keane TE, Moore RG, Lumsden AB (2003) Concomitant intraoperative renal artery embolization and resection of complex renal carcinoma. *Journal of Vascular Surgery* **38**: 446–450.

Lipponen P, Eskelinen M, Hietala K, Syrjanen K, Gambetta RA (1994) Expression of proliferating cell nuclear antigen (PC10), p53 protein and c-erbB-2 in renal adenocarcinoma. *International Journal of Cancer* **57**: 275–280.

Manke C, Bretschneider T, Lenhart M, Strotzer M, Neumann C, Gmeinwieser J et al. (2001) Spinal metastases from renal cell carcinoma: effect of preoperative particle embolization on intraoperative blood loss. *American Journal of Neuroradiology* **22**: 997–1003.

Motzer RJ, Mazumdar M, Bacik J, Berg W, Amsterdam A, Ferrara J (1999) Survival and prognostic stratification of 670 patients with advanced renal cell carcinoma. *Journal of Clinical Oncology* **17**: 2530–2540.

Motzer RJ, Mazumdar M, Bacik J et al. (2000) Effect of cytokine therapy on survival for patients with advanced renal cell carcinoma. *Journal of Clinical Oncology* **18**: 1928–1935.

Munro NP, Woodhams S, Nawrocki JD, Fletcher MS, Thomas PJ (2003) The role of transarterial embolization in the treatment of renal cell carcinoma. *BJU International* **92**: 240–244.

Onufrey V & Mohiuddin M (1985) Radiation therapy in the treatment of metastatic renal cell carcinoma. *International Journal of Radiation Oncology, Biology, Physics* **11**: 2007–2009.

Papadopoulos I, Rudolph P, Weichert-Jacobsen K, Thiemann O, Papadopoulou D (1996) Prognostic indicators for response to therapy and survival in patients with metastatic renal cell cancer treated with interferon alpha-2 beta and vinblastine. *Urology* **48**: 373–378.

Patchell R, Tibbs PA, Regine WF, Payne R, Saris S, Kryscio RJ, Young B (2003) A randomized trial of direct decompressive surgical resection in the treatment of spinal cord compression caused by metastasis. *Proceedings of the American Society of Clinical Oncology* **22**: 1.

Ro JY, Ayala AG, Sella A, Samuels ML, Swanson DA (1987) Sarcomatoid renal cell carcinoma: clinicopathologic. A study of 42 cases. *Cancer* **59**: 516–526.

Sella A, Logothetis CJ, Ro JY, Swanson DA, Samuels ML (1987) Sarcomatoid renal cell carcinoma. A treatable entity. *Cancer* **60**: 1313–1318.

Tannapfel A, Hahn HA, Katalinic A, Fietkau RJ, Kuhn R, Wittekind CW (1996) Prognostic value of ploidy and proliferation markers in renal cell carcinoma. *Cancer* **77**: 164–171.

Wilson D, Hiller L, Gray L, Grainger M, Stirling AJ, James N (2003) The effect of radiotherapy dose in the palliation of symptomatic metastatic renal cell carcinoma. *Clinical Oncology.* (In the press.)

Zisman A, Pantuck AJ, Dorey F et al. (2001) Improved prognostication of renal cell carcinoma using an integrated staging system. *Journal of Clinical Oncology* **19**: 1649–1657.

PART 5

Management of metastases

Chapter 13

The surgical management of spinal metastases from renal cell carcinoma

Alistair J Stirling, Andrew M McGee and Mel F Grainger

Introduction

Incidence and consequence

In 1995, 5557 new cases of renal cell carcinoma (RCC) were diagnosed in the UK. It accounts for only 3% of all malignancies, although two-thirds will develop skeletal metastases and 60% of these will develop within 3 months of initial diagnosis (Durr et al. 1999). Spinal metastases develop in up to 50% and nearly half of these occur within 3 months (Tatsui et al. 1996). It is the fourth most common tumour to metastasise to the spine and the most common cause of neurological compression in those presenting with unknown primaries (Schaberg and Gainor 1985). Spinal renal metastases often result in pathological vertebral collapse, causing disabling pain that is difficult to control. Paresis or paralysis often follows or may be the presenting feature. Untreated, high levels of dependency result in high financial and human costs. Renal metastases are relatively radioresistant and surgical treatment is often indicated. There appears to be an increasing incidence of renal metastases but an improving prognosis over the last 30 years (McLaughlin and Lipworth 2000; Pantuck et al. 2001). The aggressive surgical treatment of spinal metastases practised in some countries may have contributed to the improved prognosis.

Historical background

Historically surgical management of spinal metastatic disease was considered inappropriate because, before the introduction of modern oncological treatments, the overall prognosis for most of these patients was poor.

Early surgery was limited to decompressive laminectomy to prevent or treat neurological compromise. However, this failed either to address the instability of the anterior column (vertebral body) or to provide adequate anterior decompression of the cord. This resulted in poor neurological recovery and persistent pain (Merrin et al. 1976; Liskow et al. 1986). Radiotherapy combined with steroids was demonstrated to be at least as effective as laminectomy (Findlay 1984), making surgery difficult to justify. Spinal instrumentation primarily developed for correction of spinal deformity (e.g. the Harrington rod and the Hartshill rectangle) was then used in an attempt to improve stability, but being intended for use with an intact anterior spinal column it proved inadequate. Over the past two decades, there has been considerable improvement in the spinal constructs available to manage spinal structural deficiency. Concurrently, adjuvant methods of oncological treatment have improved significantly such that surgery to prevent or reverse neurological compromise, or to treat disabling pain from instability, has become a justifiable consideration.

General medical awareness

Despite the advances in oncology and spinal surgery, there remains a low level of awareness in the general medical community, in both hospital and primary care setting, of what can be achieved. A recent review of patients with breast cancer documented that, in only 45 of 207 with painful skeletal metastases and in only 6 of 51 patients with spinal instability, was orthopaedic opinion sought (Galasko et al. 2000).

A similar review by O'Donoghue documented that, in only half the instances where an orthopaedic review was indicated, was this undertaken and only 50% of suitable patients were operated upon. The authors concluded that there was a lack of awareness of the treatment possibilities by both oncologists and non-spinal orthopaedic surgeons alike, and also that there was a failure of postgraduate courses and 'broad-spectrum' journals to highlight the problems of spinal instability associated with metastases. Other series have showed rates of referral as low as 3.4–6.4% (Tatsui et al. 1996; Jackson et al. 2001).

Literature review and evidence levels

There is no prospective randomised controlled trial (RCT) in the literature. It would probably be unethical to undertake an RCT given the historical experience of failure to stabilise the spine in the presence of pathological failure and/or neurological compromise.

Dedicated series of spinal renal metastases

We have found only two papers focusing solely on surgical treatment of renal metastases to the spine, although there are numerous other papers on spinal metastases that include renal carcinoma.

King et al. (1991) reported on the surgical treatment of 33 renal cell spinal metastases. The average age was 55 (range 22–72) years. They performed 21 anterior, 9 posterior and 3 combined surgical procedures, depending on the location of the tumour, using a variety of instrumentation in 29 patients. Relief of pain occurred in 29 (88%) and 12 of the 20 (60%) improved neurologically (10 improving one Frankel grade – Frankerl et al. 1969). Overall survival was 8 months but 11 patients survived over 10 months and 6 patients survived more than 2 years. Survival did not correlate with age or time since nephrectomy. Patients who had one operation survived an average of 6 months compared with 15 months for those who required further surgery. This was thought to reflect the general health of the patient, although it may indicate differing patterns of tumour behaviour. Symptomatic recurrence in 16 (49%) developed at a mean of 5.2 months and was not affected by pre- or postoperative radiotherapy. Nine underwent further surgery; the remaining seven were unfit for further intervention.

Jackson et al. (2001) recently reported 79 patients with renal spinal metastases. A total of 103 procedures were performed for significant pain in 88% and/or neurological compromise in 51%. The mean follow-up was 10 months in those who died and 23 months in those still surviving. The nature of the procedure was dependent on the location of the metastasis, with attempted fusion in all with tumour-related instability. Half the patients received preoperative embolisation, but intraoperative blood loss did not differ between those who were embolised and those who were not. Forty patients had preoperative radiotherapy and 70 received either pre- or postoperative immuno- or chemotherapy; 46% had posterior surgery, 32% anterior surgery and 24% combined procedures. Out of 55 patients with preoperative neurological deficit 36 improved, but only 22 patients changed their Frankel grading. Two patients deteriorated neurologically after surgery. Postoperatively, pain levels improved significantly, although greater relief was seen with longer survival. The postoperative survival was 12.3 months with a 5-year survival rate predicted at 15%. There was a 15% incidence of major complications.

We have reviewed our own experience of metastatic RCC to the spine. Of 27 surgical patients, 15 were patients in whom the metastasis was the first presentation of disease. Of those with previously diagnosed disease, the mean interval to presentation with spinal metastasis was 30.3 months (range 1–201). Although those with known disease were identified earlier (11.7 weeks vs 17.1 weeks), this did not reach statistical significance. Twelve patients had neurological symptoms at presentation, although only ten had demonstrable neurological deficit (two were Frankel grade C). Eleven patients had single level disease, of whom four had posterior, three anterior and four combined procedures. Of the remaining sixteen patients, ten had posterior, four combined and two anterior procedures. Only one patient was not stabilised and 15 patients had attempted fusion. Survival at 6 months was 59%, at 12 months 36% and at 36 months 27%. Pain was improved in most patients. Four patients deteriorated neurologically after surgery, one 3 weeks postoperatively with an anterior spinal artery thrombosis who had previously had high-dose radiotherapy. A second had progression of disease at a higher level, with the general condition preventing further surgery. Only one lost the ability to walk. Of those with a preoperative neurological deficit 50% improved 1 Frankel grade. The mean Karnofsky performance score (Karnofsky 1967) improved from 61.9 preoperatively to 70.0 postoperatively. Three patients required four subsequent procedures two at the same level (2 weeks and 14 months postoperatively) and two at different levels (2 months and 4 months). There were five wound-related problems, one temporary brachial plexus palsy and two chest infections.

General series of spinal metastases

Papers including renal tumours in their data have been summarised in Table 13.1. Given the differing indications, and limited information on spread, neurology and treatments for individual tumours, only general conclusions can be reached. The number of patients presenting with spinal metastasis as a first manifestation of malignancy ranged from 7% to 40% (Tatsui et al. 1996; Klekamp and Samii 1998; Durr et al. 1999), although our own series is higher than this (56%). The indications for spinal surgery cited were failure of non-operative treatment, pain unresponsive to analgesia, neurological deterioration, spinal instability and vertebral collapse. Various methods of stabilisation have been utilised including:

- Anterior decompression with instrumentation using polymethylmethacrylate cement (PMMA) or bone graft with Steinmann pins, rods, plate and screws, ceramic or metal cages.
- Posterior decompression with instrumentation using Luque rods, Hartshill rectangle or pedicle screw fixation systems.
- Total spondylectomy for extralesional excisions (Tomita et al. 1994; Sundaresan et al. 1989; Abe et al. 2000).

Preoperative embolisation of renal metastases was performed on some but not all patients. Survival rates published vary and, given the lack of standardisation of the patients, it is difficult to draw many conclusions. In the combined series renal metastasis made up approximately 12.7% (range 1.7–32.9) of all cases (Manabe et al. 1989; King et al. 1991; Kocialkowski and Webb 1992; Jónsson et al. 1994, 1996; Hosono et al. 1995; Onimus et al. 1996; Bauer 1997; Enkaoua et al. 1997; Nazarian et al. 1997; Turgut et al. 1997; Gokaslan et al. 1998; Weigel et al. 1999; Wise et al. 1999; Abe et al. 2000; Bilsky et al. 2000; Chataigner and Onimus 2000; Chen et al. 2000; Jackson et al. 2001).

Survival was quoted by Kaplan–Meier's method or by the mean. Mean survival period was quoted by either time to death, survival in those still alive or the mean for the whole cohort. Despite this, two features can be identified. Mean survival overall appears to be around 12 months with a 25–30% survival rate at 3 years. Perhaps more interesting is the pattern of deaths. Jackson et al. (2001) and our own series have found a cohort who die in less than a year after surgery, but another group who survive much longer, typically in excess of 2 years. This suggests a bimodal pattern of survival and is supported by the findings of Tatsui et al. (1996). In those with longer survival the tumour appears to be less aggressive even with other metastases present. Improved understanding of an individual tumour (RCC) will help in anticipating the likely prognosis and thereby the appropriate scale and type of spinal surgical procedure(s) required.

Table 13.1 Review of experience in the surgical treatment of renal metastases to the spine

Study	No of renal patients	Neurological outcome	Survival (months)	Complication rate (%)	No requiring further surgery	Comments
Jackson et al. (2000)	79	22/55 improved, 1 Frankel grade, 2 deteriorated	12.3 months mean, 15.3%, 5 years	15	19	Embolisation associated with 8.5% rate of neurological deterioration Mean survival 10 months deceased, 23 months surviving
King et al. (1991)	33	50% improved 1 Frankel grade	8 months mean, 33% > 10m, 6/33 > 2years	Not available	9/33	
Present series	27	5/10 improved 1 Frankel	13.5 mean, 59% 6 months, 36% 12 months, 27% 36 months	8/27	3/27	Survival 8.0 months for deceased, 34.4 months surviving patients
Durr et al. (1999)	15/45	Recovery in 5/15 not quoted 3 deteriorated	49% 1 year, 39% 2 year, 25% 3 year, 28% 5 year with single metastasis	8/45	Not available	No difference in outcome between axial & appendicular skeleton
Sioutos et al. (1995)	15/109	9/39 in whole group regained ambulation	Mean 20.9 months (range 6–84)	17	7/15	11% surgical mortality rate
Wise et al. (1999)	6/80	19/38 improved 1 Frankel grade	11.3 months mean	100	8/80	Mean survival from diagnosis of spinal met 18 months. 2.3% 30-day mortality rate, 2 neurological deteriorations with surgery
Tatsui et al. (1996)	29/425	Not recorded in 5 patients operated	51.2% 6 and 12 months 39.5% 36 months (from detection of spinal metastasis)	Not available	0	In 5 operated patients, survival 22.6 months (1–46)
Klekamp and Samii (1998)	12/106	22% of whole group regained	46.5% 1 year all patients	16	Not available	6 month survival 70.9% ability to walk for elective procedures and 53.9 for emergency

As treatment is for the most part palliative, quality of life is paramount. The literature supports spinal surgery as being helpful to many patients in this respect. Weigel et al. (1999) found 80% of patients undergoing anterior surgery who were satisfied or very satisfied with their surgery and two-thirds achieved moderate or good health as assessed by the Karnofsky index. Similarly, Chataigner and Onimus (2000) found 'surgery in vertebral metastasis without neurological deficit results in substantial functional improvement'. Neurological recovery in many series was disappointing with recovery of 1 Frankel grade by only 22–50% (King et al. 1991; Sioutos et al. 1995; Klekamp and Samii 1998; Wise et al. 1999; Jackson et al. 2001). None of these reports relates recovery to duration of neurological deficit. Neurological deterioration after surgery was 2.5–20% (Durr et al. 1999; Wise et al. 1999; Jackson et al. 2001).

Local recurrence rates were high, reflecting the low radiosensitivity of renal metastases and that most excisions were intralesional. Information on the time to local recurrence and the number requiring further operations is scant. Nazarian et al. (1997) reported a disease-free period of 7 months but does not state how many became symptomatic or the number requiring further operations. Abe et al. (2000) performed extralesional excisions of single metastasis in two patients but had a 100% recurrence rate.

Assessment of the patient

Presentation

This is generally in one or more of the following modes.

Back pain in isolation

In some it may be apparent that symptoms are similar to previous episodes of degenerative origin. In others new pain of a mechanical type may be suggestive of a pathological fracture. In either instance neurological examination must be performed. It is suggested that plain radiographs should be obtained in all those with a history of malignancy and recent onset of spinal pain. Whole-spine sagittal magnetic resonance imaging (MRI) would ideally be performed but availability and cost preclude this at present.

Incipient neurological compromise

All patients with partial neurological deficit should be assumed to be at risk of sudden deterioration, and should be referred to a spinal surgeon. MRI should be performed.

Complete neurological deficit

If gradual in onset and within hours of becoming complete, surgery may be considered. If rapid in onset or with complete deficit of more than 12 hours' duration, the probability of significant recovery, particularly in elderly people, is low.

If the pain is severe or there is a partial neurological deficit, it may be appropriate to treat the patient because there is a risk of a potentially unstable spine until imaging confirms reasonable structural integrity.

If instability is confirmed, a spinal bed is recommended (with collar if cervical) to assist in nursing before definitive management. The nursing staff require familiarity with care of patients with an unstable spine.

Patient factors

Assessment of the patient with spinal metastatic disease requires consideration of the following contributory factors.

Biological, as opposed to chronological, age is of significance in determining recovery from surgery. An assessment of general medical condition is mandatory to exclude important co-morbidity, which may prejudice the outcome. It has an important bearing on the magnitude of surgery contemplated and the approach. Also, the recovery from surgery is influenced by patient motivation.

Many of these patients are elderly and some may not wish to consider a surgical option. Sensitive discussion by the spinal surgical consultant is required with both patients and relatives about the advantages and disadvantages.

Spinal factors

It needs to be defined whether compression of the spinal cord is caused by the tumour in isolation or alternatively by a pathological fracture. If the latter, radiotherapy will not be effective and surgical decompression is mandatory to allow neurological improvement.

Accurate preoperative assessment of the degree of spinal involvement is mandatory and MRI is the gold standard. Neither the information available from the CT scan nor that from the isotope scan is adequate. Whole-spine sagittal MRI is required to determine the extent of involvement of the spinal column with axial imaging of the areas involved. In RCC bony metastatic lesions are often 'cold' on isotope scans. Computed tomography (CT) may, however, assist in defining the degree of osteolysis and areas where fixation can be achieved.

Whether compression is proximal to or distal to the conus medullaris, or whether compression is from anterior or posterior, is important in surgical planning.

The duration and degree of neurological compromise are important. With the onset of complete paresis, immediate intervention is required if neurological recovery is to be anticipated. In the presence of incomplete neurological deficit, urgent transfer to a unit equipped to assess and manage the patient at an early stage is mandatory.

Tumour factors

The subtype and grade of renal tumour and the anticipated prognosis are of prime importance and require close liaison between the spinal surgeon and oncologist.

Whether or not the tumour is sensitive to adjuvant treatment such as chemotherapy, radiotherapy or hormone manipulation is of great relevance because there is no point in utilising these modalities in the presence of actual or potential neurological compromise, unless the tumour is sensitive.

Staging to determine the extent of visceral and skeletal involvement is essential, providing the neurological status of the patient permits. This has a fundamental bearing on whether the surgery planned is curative or merely palliative.

Preoperative observation

A complete history and examination with particular attention to neurological status is mandatory. Neurological charts should be available and completed at the frequency clinically indicated and on a daily basis as a minimum. Input/output charts are needed to monitor sphincter function.

Laboratory investigations

- Haematology: blood count, erythrocyte sedimentation rate (ESR), coagulation profile
- Biochemistry: liver function tests (LFTs), bone biochemistry, renal function
- Site-dependent tumour markers.

Imaging

- MRI: whole-spine sagittal T1 and T2; axials of involved areas
- Plain radiographs of area of spine involved – define local bony anatomy for screw placement
- *Chest radiograph: whole lung CT*
- *Liver imaging: CT or ultrasonography*
- *Isotope bone scan.*

Those in italics represent desirable staging investigations and should not be allowed to delay intervention if neurology is deteriorating.

Postoperative staging will involve the histological grade of tumour and tumour-free margins.

Biopsy

It cannot be assumed that skeletal metastases are necessarily from the same primary tumour as previously treated, particularly if there has been a prolonged latent period. In a number of instances, second primary tumours have been responsible for metastatic deposits causing paresis. In our experience, 6% of patients with spinal metastasis have a second primary.

- Biopsy of an apparently solitary lesion should not be undertaken without discussion with a spinal centre.
- Biopsy usually requires imaging control in the form either of CT or biplanar image intensifier.
- Dependent upon site, this can be undertaken under local or general anaesthesia.
- It should normally be performed as a trephine.
- It should be performed only after MR images have been obtained because haemorrhage at the biopsy site may influence interpretation of the scan.

Renal metastases have the potential to be very vascular and it is recommended that the patient should have blood cross-match or at least have his or her serum group assessed and saved before biopsy. Similarly, it is possible that biopsy may result in haemorrhage within the spinal canal, with rapid neurological compromise; facilities should be available to proceed to urgent decompression if required.

Scoring systems

Two scoring systems to identify which patients should be considered for spinal surgery have been reported. At this time only the Tokuhashi Score (Tokuhashi et al. 1990) has been independently validated. Our data support both systems (Grainger et al. 2002). The Tokuhashi Score is more comprehensive and includes the Karnofsky performance score (Karnofsky 1967), number of extraspinal metastases, number of vertebral metastases, visceral metastases, primary tumour type and presence of neurological deficit. The Tomita Score (Tomita et al. 2001) includes type of primary tumour, visceral metastases and bone metastases. Neither of these systems is designed to give a prognosis, but to direct the type of spinal surgery for which the patient may be suitable (extralesional or marginal excision, intralesional excision or stabilisation, or palliation only). To this end they form a useful guide.

Treatment selection

Radiotherapy

Radiotherapy or chemotherapy might be considered if there is no pathological fracture or spinal instability and if cord compression is the result of tumour rather than retropulsed bone, without clinically significant neurological deficit, and the tumour is thought to be sensitive. Other indications include multilevel disease, stable or slowly progressive deteriorating neurology, poor prognosis and poor general condition. Adjuvant radiotherapy may be used for local control after surgery

Surgery

In most, the objective of surgery is palliation. In the small minority in whom there appears to be a truly isolated secondary and the situation permits, the objective may be attempted curative resection. Ideally this would be performed as an extralesional resection. Given the frequent involvement of both anterior and posterior columns, *de facto* intralesional resection is the best that can be achieved.

Palliative surgery is indicated where there is intractable pain unresponsive to non-operative measures or insensitive to adjuvant treatment, spinal instability (evidenced by pathological fracture, progressive deformity and/or neurological deficit) or clinically significant neurological compression, and patients who have reached the limit of spinal cord tolerance after prior radiotherapy.

Operative aspects

The objectives of surgery are to maintain or restore the function of the spinal cord and nerve roots. It should restore mechanical stability of the vertebral column if compromised and should aim to preserve as many normal motion segments as possible. Ideally, either anterior or posterior surgery alone should be sufficient to provide adequate decompression and stability. The magnitude of the procedure should not exceed the patient's ability to survive it or the surgeon's level of competence to execute it.

Embolisation

Preoperative embolisation is normally performed because metastases are usually very vascular (Chuang et al. 1979) and excision may lead to massive blood loss and/or postoperative haematoma with potential neurological compromise (Olerud et al. 1993). Preoperative embolisation significantly reduces blood loss (Rowe et al. 1984; Roscoe et al. 1989; Gellad et al. 1990; Olerud et al. 1993; Hess et al. 1997), improving visibility during surgery, and may reduce the risk of exsanguination and/or postoperative haematoma. Embolisation is not without risk and severe neurological deficit has been reported (Gokaslan et al. 1998; Jackson et al. 2001). Careful consideration is required if major spinal cord feeding vessels are to be embolised (especially the Adamkiewicz (1882) artery). It is recommended, however, that whenever possible embolisation should be performed before surgery.

Facilities

In the presence of significant neurological compromise, recognition of the surgical priority of many of these cases is required and may require displacement of other less pressing cases. Ideally, however, surgery should be performed during normal hours with full support.

Clean air operating facilities should be used whenever possible. Spinal operating tables are required, permitting biplanar imaging.

Operating theatre staff need to be familiar with the approaches and instrumentation proposed.

Surgical exposure

The surgeon requires familiarity with anterior and posterior approaches to all spinal levels. Junctional areas (occipitocervical, cervicothoracic, lumbosacral) require particular experience and often specialised approaches, and may need referral to specialised centres.

Decompression and stabilisation

Except in very unusual circumstances, decompression should not be undertaken without adjunctive stabilisation.

The direction of neurological compression is important in surgical planning. Usually, if compression is anterior, an anterior approach is preferable, but co-morbidity may dictate opting for a posterior approach. Posterior or posterolateral decompression for anterior compression is more difficult, particularly proximal to the conus, and less likely to be complete. Distal to the conus medullaris, satisfactory posterior decompression can be performed more safely for either posterior or anterior compression.

The surgeon should be familiar with use of the instrumentation intended in non-pathological bone. More significant technical challenges can be posed, given the variable quality of the bone encountered in the pathological situation.

- Implants should provide immediate stability to facilitate early mobilisation.
- Anterior constructs should be sufficiently strong not to require additional posterior support. Posterior fixation is not required as long as the posterior elements remain competent.
- Posterior constructs should be rectangular for maximal stability. Pedicle screw-based systems provide maximum purchase while instrumenting the minimum number of segments. Screw purchase can be enhanced by injection of bone cement into the pedicle before screw insertion, although the possibility of cement leaking into the canal makes this an uncommon practice.
- Implants should be titanium, permitting later repeat MRI if necessary.
- A full range of implants for anterior and posterior reconstruction at all levels is required 'in house'.

Fusion

If the prognosis exceeds 6 months, it is probably advisable to consider synchronous fusion to avoid possible failure of the implant or at the bone–implant interface.

Postoperative requirements

Postoperative care is as important as the surgery. Maintenance of circulation and oxygenation are essential to maintain optimum perfusion to the spinal cord. Neurology should be recorded at the end of the procedure, and documented hourly in a high-dependency unit postoperatively. If patients are unable to urinate, perineal sensation and anal tone should be assessed to exclude incipient cord compromise caused by haematoma. Neurological deterioration mandates an emergency MRI and/or re-exploration.

Complications

Complication rates for tumour surgery are higher than for other types of spinal surgery. Infection is an avoidable disaster, although rates vary from 16% to 100% (Sioutos et al. 1995; Klekamp and Samii 1998; Durr et al. 1999; Wise et al. 1999; Jackson et al. 2001). Wherever possible a clean air operating theatre should be used and antibiotic prophylaxis should be given. These patients are at particular risk of thromboembolism. This has to balance against the potential risk of chemical prophylaxis causing haemorrhage and neural compression. As a minimum, mechanical prophylaxis is recommended.

Adjuvant therapies

It is important to re-emphasise that, in the presence of spinal instability, consequent upon pathological fracture with or without neurological compromise, the primary task is the re-establishment of spinal stability and, if necessary, decompression of the neural elements. This is necessarily a surgical task.

It should be recognized that, in most metastatic disease, it is very unusual for truly isolated secondary disease to be present. This does, however, appear to occur more frequently with renal disease than with other tumours. If this is thought to be present, it may be justifiable to attempt a radical clearance of the disease, if the general condition of the patient permits, in the hope of improving prognosis.

In most circumstances patients have multiple metastases and subtotal clearance of tumour with adequate decompression and stabilisation is the surgical goal. Control of remaining disease is dependent on the appropriate adjuvant therapies.

In general, decisions as to the timing and type of adjuvant therapy should be made jointly with the site-specific specialist and oncologist/radiotherapist. In broad terms, an adequate period should be allowed for skin healing and if fusion has been performed for the initial phases of bone healing. There remains some dispute as to how long it is necessary to delay radiotherapy so that it does not interfere with bone healing.

Cost–benefits and implications

In deciding whether surgical management is appropriate, important considerations are whether the patient will benefit in relief of distress caused by pain, relief of disability resulting from neurological deficit and the recovery period from surgery relative to their overall prognosis. It is also important whether society will benefit in terms of both the cost of the procedure and the evolution of new treatment methods.

In 1995, the costs of posterior surgery including the inpatient stay were assessed at £7600 per patient on average (Birmingham). Previous studies in Nottingham and Upsala have demonstrated that the cost of surgical intervention is lower than conservative care if patient survival exceeds 8 weeks in Sweden or 10 weeks in Nottingham.

Provision of an adequate assessment and treatment service for these patients would impose significant increased demands on both orthopaedic and neurosurgical services. There would also be significantly increased demand for imaging services

Inadequate primary surgery may result in a requirement for revision surgery. In addition to the costs involved, this will normally impinge significantly upon the patients' remaining life expectancy. It normally results from:

- Patients outliving their anticipated prognosis and accordingly the estimated longevity of construct employed.
- Failure to employ a sufficiently biomechanically robust construct in the initial instance.
- Using posterior constructs in isolation in those with a long prognosis.

Awareness of surgical intervention

All patients with renal carcinoma should be made aware of the possibility of bony metastases as part of their initial education. On development of symptoms suggestive of bony metastases, they should have clear instructions about from whom to seek further advice (this will vary locally and needs to be defined.).

Experience continues to confirm that these patients may not be adequately advised in the primary care setting and timely access to specialist opinion and investigation is imperative. Improved education of the primary care sector is a priority, particularly given their current increased responsibility for the rationing of health care.

Even in the hospital sector there remains a low level of awareness of the level of development of spinal reconstructive techniques and when these can be applicable. It is suggested that all patients in whom there is a question about the feasibility of reconstruction should have a consultant spinal surgical opinion before this is dismissed. Many patients with isolated spinal metastasis without visceral involvement may well have a reasonable prognosis given adequate treatment of their spinal disease.

Organisational aspects

Despite the Calman initiative in the recognition of site-specific oncology services, there has been a singular failure to recognise the final common pathway of many patients with spinal metastatic disease and to define adequate levels of provision of service and appropriate funding. As with the appendicular skeleton the management of spinal metastases is currently subject to widely variable practice. In some areas there is no clearly defined separate service or on-call responsibility for reconstructive spinal surgery, the requirements for which are quite different to those of decompressive spinal surgery. There are approximately 50 orthopaedic and 15 neurosurgical consultants who are full-time spinal surgeons. There are an additional 148 orthopaedic surgeons with a major interest in spinal surgery and 165 neurosurgeons, most of whom will undertake some spinal procedures. It is not clear how many of either have the experience or facilities to undertake procedures of this nature.

Within each health region, clear definition of those responsible for the provision of service for reconstructive spinal surgery is required. It is anticipated that this will normally be the remit of those charged with provision of service for patients with spinal trauma and infection, because the requirements are broadly similar. There needs to be a clear central recognition of the level of facility required for provision of this service, and it should be appropriately financed.

Appropriate audit of referral, surgical requirement and outcome should be compiled and made available for national comparison. In particular, details of those in whom no intervention is undertaken and the reasons for this should be included. Financial and administrative support for this should be made available.

Within each district general hospital (DGH), it is recommended that an individual should have the responsibility for the development and supervision of a suitable assessment and care pathway. Given that most DGHs have an in-house orthopaedic service and that assessment of both the appendicular and axial skeleton should normally be within their ability, it is suggested that this would form the basis of the initial assessment.

It is recommended that organisation of a reconstructive spinal service should be regarded as the equivalent of one clinical session. It is anticipated that this will include development of appropriate links with the urologist and oncologists/radiotherapists. It would also include definition by local and mutual agreement of the route and clinical content of referral. In some areas, and where demand is sufficient, a clinic dedicated to this purpose may be appropriate.

It is imperative that sufficient and timely access to the appropriate imaging facilities is made available, notwithstanding that this may mean significant alteration to current custom and practice in on-call availability. With the recent provision of MRI facilities in most DGHs, it is no longer acceptable to transfer patients in pain and at peril of neurological deterioration to a centre for consideration of surgery, only to return them to the referring DGH when it has become apparent that there is no surgical option.

Conclusions and recommendations

Spinal metastases from renal carcinoma are common, and frequently cause pain and/or neurological compromise. Although curative surgery for isolated spinal metastasis remains unproven, the 5-year life expectancies being obtained in some centres make aggressive surgery a consideration. In patients with more widespread disease, symptom control and quality of life can be significantly improved, if not the overall prognosis. Recovery of neurological deficit is unpredictable but less likely if onset is rapid and decompression is not done early. Identification of patients with spinal metastasis at an early stage does not necessitate early surgical intervention, but should stimulate dialogue between oncologists and spinal surgeons to promote individualised solutions for each patient. Surgical treatment and radiotherapy are complementary and not competitive. If oncologists can control the disease, spinal surgeons can now often control the spine.

Education of what can be achieved for many of these patients remains a priority. The spinal surgical community needs to heighten the awareness of professional colleagues in both primary and secondary care of the possibilities that exist. Patients should be aware at the outset of their disease about the possibility of spinal involvement and that this can often be addressed to good effect. Early consultation with time for a considered decision is clearly preferable to urgent unplanned surgery. The painful paralysis associated with spinal metastatic disease is now often avoidable.

References

Abe E, Sato K, Murai H, Tazawa H, Chiba M, Okuyama K (2000) Total spondylectomy for solitary spinal metastasis of the thoracolumbar spine: A preliminary report. *Tohoku Journal of Experimental Medicine* **190**: 33–49.

Adamkiewicz A (1882) Die Blutgefasse des menschlichen Rückenmarkes. Tiel II. Die Gefesse der Rückenmarks-Oberfläche. *Sitzungsberichte der Kaiserlichen Akademie der Wissenschaften, Mathematischnatur-Wissenschaftliche Classe, Wien* **85**: 101–130.

Bauer HCF (1997) Posterior decompression and stabilization for spinal metastases. *Journal of Bone and Joint Surgery* **79A**: 514–522.

Bilsky MH, Boland P, Lis E, Raizer JJ, Healey JH (2000) Single-stage posterolateral transpedicle approach for spondylectomy, epidural decompression, and circumferential fusion of spinal metastases. *Spine* **25**: 2240–2250.

Chataigner H, Onimus M (2000) Surgery in spinal metastasis without spinal cord compression: indications and strategy related to the risk of recurrence. *European Spine Journal* **9**: 523–527.

Chen LH, Chen WJ, Niu CC, Shih CH (2000) Anterior reconstructive spinal surgery with Zielke instrumentation for metastatic malignancies of the spine. *Archives of Orthopedic and Trauma Surgery* **120**: 27–31.

Chuang VP, Wallace S, Swanson D et al. (1979) Arterial occlusion in the management of pain from metastatic renal carcinoma. *Radiology* **133**: 611–614.

Durr HR, Maier M, Pfahler M, Baur A, Refior HJ (1999) Surgical treatment of osseous metastases in patients with renal cell carcinoma. *Clinical Orthopaedics* **367**: 282–290.

Enkaoua EA, Doursounian L, Chatellier G, Mabesoone F, Aimard T, Saillant G (1997) Vertebral metastases: a critical appreciation of the preoperative prognostic Tokuhashi score in a series of 71 cases. *Spine* **22**: 2293–2298.

Findlay GF (1984) Adverse effects of the management of malignant spinal cord compression. *Journal of Neurology, Neurosurgery, and Psychiatry* **47**: 761–768.

Frankel HL, Hancock DO, Hyslop G et al. (1969) The value of postural reduction in the initial management of closed injuries of the spine with paraplegia and tetraplegia. *Paraplegia* **7**: 179–192.

Galasko CSB, Norris HE, Crank S (2000) Spinal instability secondary to metastatic cancer. *Journal of Bone and Joint Surgery* **82A**: 570–577.

Gellad FE, Sadato N, Numaguchi Y, Levine AM (1990) Vascular metastatic lesions of the spine: preoperative embolization. *Radiology* **176**: 683–686.

Gokaslan ZL, York JE, Walsh GL et al. (1998) Transthoracic vertebrectomy for metastatic spinal tumors. *Journal of Neurosurgery* **89**: 599–609.

Grainger MF, Stirling AJ, Marks DS, Thompson AG, Jackowski A (2002) Validation of two prognostic scoring systems used in the treatment of spinal metastases. Presented at Britspine 2002, 27 Feb–1 March, Birmingham, UK.

Hess T, Kramann B, Schmidt E, Rupp S (1997) Use of preoperative vascular embolisation in spinal metastasis resection. *Archives of Orthopaedic Trauma* **116**: 279–282.

Hosono N, Yonenobu K, Fuji T, Ebara S, Yamashita K, Ono K (1995) Vertebral body replacement with a ceramic prosthesis for metastatic spinal tumours. *Spine* **20**: 2454–2462.

Jackson RJ, Gokaslan ZL, Loh SC (2001) Metastatic renal cell carcinoma of the spine: surgical treatment and results. *Journal of Neurosurgery* **94**(suppl 1): 18–24.

Jónsson B, Jónsson H Jr, Karlström G, Sjöström L (1994) Surgery of the cervical spine metastases: a retrospective study. *European Spine Journal* **3**: 76–83.

Jónsson B, Sjöström L, Olerud C, Andréasson I, Bring J, Rauschning W (1996) Outcome after limited posterior spinal surgery for thoracic and lumbar spine metastases. *European Spine Journal* **5**: 36–44.

Karnofsky DA (1967) Clinical evaluation of anticancer drugs: cancer chemotherapy. *Gann Monographs* **2**: 223–231.

King GJ, Kostuik JP, McBroom RJ, Richardson W (1991) Surgical management of metastatic renal cell carcinoma of the spine. *Spine* **16**: 265–271.

Klekamp J, Samii H (1998) Surgical results for spinal metastases. *Acta Neurochirurgica* **140**: 957–967.

Kocialkowski A, Webb JK (1992) Metastatic spinal tumours: survival after surgery. *European Spine Journal* **1**: 43–48.

Liskow A, Chang CH, DeSanctis P, Benson M, Fetell M, Housepian E (1986) Epidural cord compression in association with genitourinary neoplasms. *Cancer* **58**: 949–954.

Manabe S, Tateishi A, Abe M, Ohno T (1989) Surgical treatment of metastatic tumors of the spine. *Spine* **14**: 41–47.

McLaughlin JK, Lipworth L (2000) Epidemiological aspects of renal cell carcinoma. *Seminars in Oncology* **27**: 115–123.

Merrin C, Avellanosa A, West C, Wajsman Z, Baumgartner G (1976) The value of palliative spinal surgery in metastatic urogenital tumours. *Journal of Urology* **115**: 712–713.

Nazarian S, Argenson C, Cordonnier D et al. (1997) Place de la chirugie dans le tratement des métastases du rachis. *Revue de Chirurgie Orthopedique* **83**(suppl 3): 109–174.

Olerud Cl, Jónsson H Jr, Löfberg A, Lörelius L, Sjöström L (1993) Embolization of spinal metastases reduces peroperative blood loss. *Acta Orthopaedica Scandinavia* **64**: 9–12.

Onimus M, Papin P, Gangloff S (1996) Results of surgical treatment of spinal thoracic and lumbar metastases. *European Spine Journal* **5**: 407–411.

Pantuck AJ, Zisman A, Belldegrun AS (2001) The changing natural history of renal cell carcinoma. *Journal of Urology* **166**: 1611–1623.

Roscoe MW, McBroom RJ, St Louis E, Grossman H, Perrin R (1989) Preoperative embolization in the treatment of osseous metastases from renal cell carcinoma. *Clinical Orthopaedics and Related Research* **238**: 302–307.

Rowe DM, Becker GJ, Rabe FE (1984) Osseous metastases from renal cell carcinoma. Embolization and surgery for restoration of function. *Radiology* **150**: 673–679.

Schaberg J, Gainor BJ (1985) A profile of metastatic carcinoma of the spine. *Spine* **10**: 19–20.

Sioutos PJ, Arbit E, Meshulam CF, Galicich JH (1995) Spinal metastases from solid tumours. Analysis of factors affecting survival. *Cancer* **76**: 1453–1459.

Sundaresan N, Di Giacinto GV, Krol G, Hughes JE (1989) Spondylectomy for malignant tumours of the spine. *Journal of Clinical Oncology* **7**: 1485–1491.

Tatsui H, Onomura T, Morishita S, Oketa M, Inoue T (1996) Survival rates of patients with metastatic spinal cancer after scintigraphic detection of abnormal radioactive accumulation. *Spine* **21**: 2143–2148.

Tokuhashi Y, Matsuzaki H, Toriyama S, Kawano H, Ohsaka S (1990) Scoring system for the preoperative evaluation of metastatic spine tumour prognosis. *Spine* **15**: 1110–1113.

Tomita K, Kawahara N, Baba H, Tsuchiya H, Nagata S, Toribatake Y (1994) Total en bloc spondylectomy for solitary spinal metastases. *International Orthopaedics* **18**: 291–298.

Tomita K, Kawahara N, Kobayashi T, Yoshida A, Murakami H, Akamuru T (2001) Surgical strategy for spinal metastases. *Spine* **26**: 298–306.

Turgut M, Gül B, Girgin O, Ta-kin Y (1997) Role of surgical treatment in 70 patients with vertebral metastasis causing cord or root compression. *Archives of Orthopedic Trauma and Surgery* **116**: 415–419.

Weigel B, Maghsudi M, Neumann C, Kretschmer R, Muller FJ, Nerlich M (1999) Surgical management of symptomatic spinal metastases. Postoperative outcome and quality of life. *Spine* **24**: 2240–2246.

Wise JJ, Fischgrund JS, Herkowitz HN, Montgomery D, Kurz KT (1999) Complications, survival rates, and risk factors of surgery for metastatic disease of the spine. *Spine* **24**: 1943–1951.

Chapter 14

Assessment and treatment of renal metastases in the pelvis and extremities

James Patton, Roger Tillman, Paul Cool and Scott Sommerville

Introduction

The five most common cancers that metastasise to bone are lung, breast, prostate, thyroid and kidney.

At the time of diagnosis, 30–60% of patients with renal cell carcinoma will have metastases (Tolia & Whitmore 1975; de Kernion et al 1978; Stener et al 1984; Maldazys & de Kernion 1986). Most of these patients will have multiple bony metastases, although 1–2% will have a solitary bony metastasis (O'Dea et al. 1978).

A recent meta-analysis of 2500 patients with metastatic bone cancer treated at five European bone tumour treatment centres included 431 patients with metastatic renal carcinoma (P Cool, unpublished data). The five-year survival of these 431 patients was 35% (Figure 14.1). Patients who had a solitary bony metastasis had a slightly better prognosis, and this has important implications for the orthopaedic management

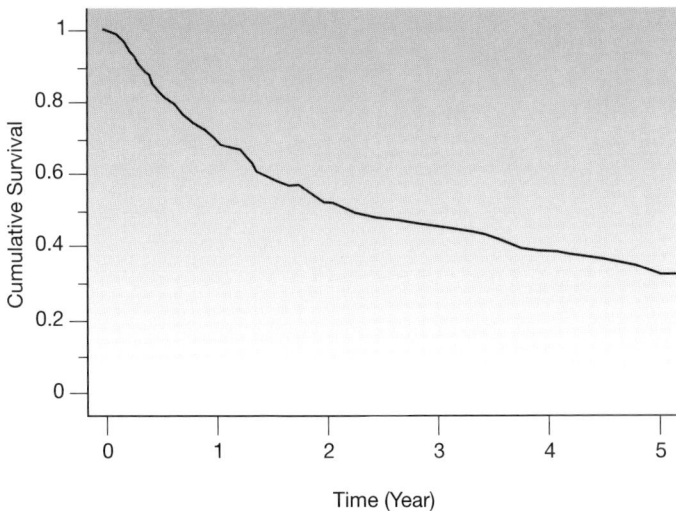

Figure 14.1 Overall survival of 431 patients with bony metastases of renal cell carcinoma. (Results of a meta-analysis of 2500 metastatic bone tumours who presented to five major bone tumour treatment centres across Europe; P Cool, unpublished data.)

(Tolia & Whitmore 1975; Middleton 1967; Montie et al. 1977; Dineen et al. 1988; Tongaonkar et al. 1992; Huguenin 1998; P Cool, unpublished data) (Figure 14.2).

The treatment of metastatic renal carcinoma is both medical and surgical and should be directed towards the primary tumour as well as the metastases. It is essential that patients are assessed by a multi-disciplinary team, so that treatment can be tailored to each individual patient's needs (Tillman 1999).

Treatment of skeletal metastases is generally palliative rather than curative. Orthopaedic treatment is aimed at preserving patients' mobility while relieving pain and preventing a pathological fracture. However, with the improvements in overall patient survival, the demands on the surgical constructs are ever-increasing.

Basic science

Malignant tumours can spread by direct extension, the lymphatic system, or through the blood stream. Haematogenous spread is the most important route in the development of bony metastases. Harrington (1988) described five steps in the process by which tumour cells spread via the blood to bone:

* release cells from the primary tumour;
* vascular invasion;

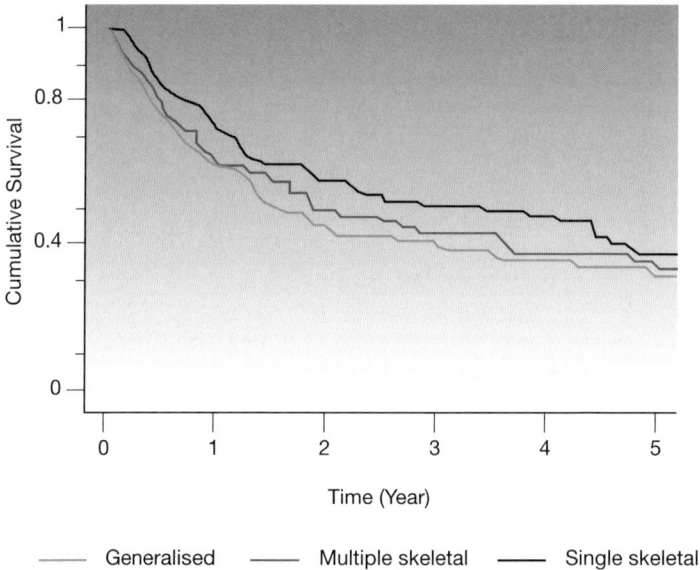

Figure 14.2 Survival of 431 patients with bony metastases of renal cell carcinoma. Patients with a solitary bony metastases have a slightly better prognosis than patients with generalised or multiple bony metastases. (Results of meta-analysis of 2500 metastatic bone tumours who presented to five major bone tumour treatment centres across Europe; P Cool, unpublished data.)

- dissemination of malignant cells via the blood;
- invasion of the bone by tumour cells;
- growth of the metastatic focus.

There are many local, systemic and tumour factors that influence these steps and the eventual development of a metastasis.

The primary tumour releases millions of cells daily into the blood stream. Only a very small proportion of these cells (0.1%) survive to establish a metastatic focus (Robbins et al. 1993), and once this distant focus becomes larger than 0.5 mm, it has to establish its own blood supply to survive.

Of importance in the dissemination of tumour cells is the paravertebral venous plexus described by Batson (Batson 1940; Robbins et al. 1993). This venous plexus extends from the skull to the sacrum and communicates with veins from the head, thorax, retro-peritoneum and proximal long bones. The veins in this plexus are valveless, which allows retrograde embolisation of tumour cells. This may explain the high incidence of metastatic deposits in the spine, pelvis, skull and proximal ends of long bones.

Metastatic deposits can be osteoblastic, osteolytic or show a mixed pattern of bone reaction. Most (84%) metastatic deposits of prostate cancer are osteoblastic, whereas renal metastases are invariably osteolytic (Capanna et al. 1999).

Renal metastases tend to be very vascular (Figure 14.3). This is related to angiogenic factors released by the tumour cells. Renal metastases also tend to expand the surrounding bone. The expansile nature of renal metastases is related to their hypervascularity; a feature they have in common with other vascular metastases such as metastatic thyroid carcinoma. If clinically palpable the metastases will often be found to be pulsatile.

Bone fractures when the stress applied to it exceeds its strength. If the bone is of abnormal strength, the fracture is called pathological. Pathological fractures occur when a bone is affected by generalised bone disease, local benign conditions, primary bone tumours or metastatic tumours. This article is only concerned with pathological fractures due to renal metastases.

It is generally accepted that osteolytic metastatic deposits have a higher chance of causing a pathological fracture (Mirels 1989).

The risk of pathological fracture is also higher in larger lesions that are located in weight-bearing bones. Clearly, the larger the lesion the more the strength of the bone is decreased. The strength of cortical bone decreases by 50% if a defect involves 50% of the intact diameter of bone, whereas it decreases by 90% if the defect involves 75% of the intact diameter (Mirels 1989; Hipp et al. 1995).

Mirels (1989) developed a scoring system to evaluate the risk of pathological fracture in a patient with a bony metastasis (Table 14.1). The scoring system is based on four parameters (site of the lesion, pain, radiological appearance and size of the

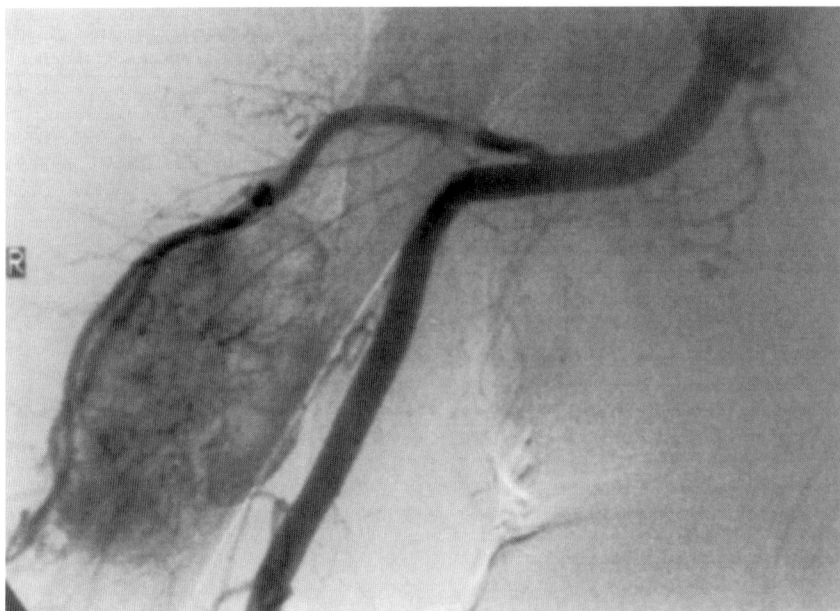

Figure 14.3 Renal metastases tend to be very vascular as is demonstrated in this angiogram. The patient had a renal secondary in the diaphysis of the humerus. Before subsequent intramedullary nailing the patient had a successful embolisation.

defect). The minimum score is 4, whereas the maximum score is 12. If the total score is higher than 8, the patient has a high risk of pathological fracture and surgical intervention to prevent pathological fracture is indicated.

It is not always easy to assess the amount of bony destruction from a standard radiograph. For an osteolytic metastasis to be visible on plain radiographs, 40% or more of the bone must have been replaced.

Computer tomography (CT) scans are more helpful in evaluating bony destruction, whereas magnetic resonance imaging (MRI) scans can be helpful to image soft-tissue involvement.

Table 14.1 Mirels (1989) scoring system to assess the risk on pathological fracture

Variable	Score		
	1	2	3
Site	Upper limb	Lower limb	Peritrochanter
Pain	Mild	Moderate	Functional
Size	< 1/3	1/3–2/3	> 2/3
Lesion	Blastic	Mixed	Lytic

Score > 8, high risk of fracture.
Score < 7, low risk of fracture.

Radioisotope bone scans are sensitive and helpful for screening purposes. High uptake of isotope indicates an increased bone turnover (such as in fractures). Renal metastases are osteolytic and often provoke only minimal reaction in the surrounding bone. A negative bone scan, therefore, does not exclude metastatic bone disease in renal carcinoma. Where pathological fracture has already occurred, the bone scan will invariably show increased uptake.

Assessment

A patient with bony metastases due to renal cell carcinoma can present in the following ways.

- Bony lesion detected at staging of renal cell carcinoma or renal cell carcinoma detected at staging of a bony lesion of previously unknown origin (synchronous metastasis).
- Bony lesion detected some time after the diagnosis of renal cell carcinoma was made (metachronous metastasis).

It is important to make this distinction, as the prognosis for synchronous metastases is worse than that of metachronous metastases (Tolia & Whitmore 1975; O'Dea et al. 1978; Pongracz et al. 1988; Baloch et al. 2000). This is presumably because, in effect, the patient is presenting with both primary tumour and metastases at the same time. The question of whether a patient with known metastases will benefit from nephrectomy to remove the primary before or after orthopaedic intervention should be discussed within the multidisciplinary team.

The prognosis in metachronous metastases is thought to be better if the disease-free interval exceeds 24 months (Middleton 1986; Tongaonkar et al. 1992).

For any symptomatic area, plain radiographs of the whole affected bone are recommended in the first instance, which can be complemented by further imaging with radioisotope bone scan, MRI, CT and angiogram as appropriate. As treatment of established disease is purely symptomatic, there is arguably no place for regular screening with repeated bone scans in the absence of symptoms.

In a patient with known renal carcinoma a lytic lesion is likely to represent a metastatic deposit, especially if there are multiple lesions. We would recommend that solitary bone lesions are investigated by appropriate imaging and bone biopsy to establish the pathology beyond any doubt. The biopsy should ideally be done by a clinician who is experienced in bone biopsies, and performed preferably by using a percutaneous technique (Mankin et al. 1982).

Clinical features

The suspicion of bone metastases will normally be raised by the onset of pain, possibly followed by a pathological fracture. Bone pain is often constant and although initially mild, it will usually gradually increase in severity. At first, pain is often unrelated to activity (i.e. non-mechanical) but typically wakes the patient at night. As the bone becomes weaker, so pain on activity becomes a more prominent and ominous feature. Back pain is, of course, common in the normal population but in the presence of known previous malignancy up to 40% of patients will be found to have metastatic disease as the cause (Galasko & Sylvester 1978).

Investigations

Phase 1

This phase should be performed in all patients with suspected metastases, and is normally completed within 24 hours (Cool & Grimer 2000). It consists of:

- history, including family history, risk factors and current symptoms;
- complete physical examination;
- blood tests, including full blood count, ESR, full biochemical and bone profile, calcium and myeloma screen;
- radiographs of the bony lesion, and entire affected bone;
- radiographs of the chest.

Phase 2

This phase consists of tests that are performed on indication and can normally be completed within a week (Cool & Grimer 2000). It may consist of:

- bone scan;
- ultrasound scan of the abdomen;
- CT scan of the chest;
- CT scan of the abdomen.

Phase 3

Phase three is usually completed by the centre treating the bone tumour. It may consist of:

- CT scan of the lesion;
- MRI scan of the lesion;
- angiogram (especially for proximal lesions);
- biopsy.

Close collaboration between pathologist, radiologist, oncologist, urologist and orthopaedic oncologist is essential in making an accurate assessment of the patient, and planning appropriate treatment.

It is important to establish:

- an estimate of the survival of the patient;
- whether the lesion is single or multiple;
- the site and extent of the lesion;
- the risk of pathological fracture.

Aims of treatment

The aim of orthopaedic treatment is to preserve the patient's mobility and function, while relieving pain and preventing pathological fracture. Surgical treatment of spinal metastases is normally done by spinal surgeons, whereas the treatment of extremity and pelvic metastases is done by orthopaedic oncologists.

It is important to note that treatment of metastases is unlikely to significantly prolong life but is aimed at improving the quality of life for the patient for whatever time remains. Any operative intervention should therefore achieve rapid restoration of function, be relatively free of complications, and, most importantly of all, should outlast the patient.

Another aspect of management is the prevention of pathological fracture. Accurately quantifying the risk of fracture in any given metastatic deposit is notoriously difficult. However, Mirels (1989) has developed a scoring system, which has been shown to be accurate at identifying those lesions that are likely to lead to fracture.

Treatment

After full multidisciplinary assessment, a treatment plan can be made. Treatment of metastatic renal cell carcinoma consists of both medical and surgical treatment.

Medical treatment

Patients who have metastatic bone cancer are frequently in pain. Early and appropriate pain relief is required while the patient is assessed and investigated. This can usually be done with a combination of analgesia, local blocks and external splintage. Symptoms and signs of hypercalcaemia should be actively looked for and treated accordingly with rehydration, diuretics and bisphosphonates.

Early involvement of an oncologist is essential. The oncologist will be able to advise on further investigations and non-surgical management. However, renal cell metastases respond relatively poorly to both chemotherapy and radiotherapy, particularly when there is extensive bone lysis, and so it cannot be assumed that any lytic lesion will consolidate. It is highly unlikely that a lesion with an established pathological fracture will unite. Therefore, surgical stabilisation of skeletal metastases remains the mainstay of treatment (Harrington 1988; Cool & Grimer 2000).

Surgical Treatment

General principles

Surgical stabilisation of skeletal metastases can be considered once the patient has been fully assessed and stabilised. It is important to have an idea of the patient's expected survival, as this will influence the method of stabilisation or reconstruction. Surgery must address the following issues.

1. The procedure must aim at relieving pain, and preserving or restoring function.
2. Recovery after surgery should be swift, allowing a rapid return to normal activities.
3. The procedure should have a low rate of complications.
4. The implant should outlast the patient.

There are three main categories of surgical treatment available.

1. Curettage of the lesion followed by internal fixation augmented with poly-methylmethacrylate cement.
2. *En bloc* excision of the affected bone/joint, usually followed by endoprosthetic replacement.
3. Amputation.

Curettage, internal fixation and cement augmentation is currently the most common method of treating skeletal metastases. The implants are readily available and relatively inexpensive. However, Wedin et al. (1999) have shown a failure rate of internal fixation of 45% in patients with renal metastases who survived for more than two years. Internal fixation implants are usually designed as load sharing devices. Their use in metastatic pathological fractures may be acceptable in the short term for patients with a short life expectancy. However, patients who may survive longer than two years may benefit from proper oncological clearance of the metastasis with *en bloc* excision and endoprosthetic replacement, especially in patients with a solitary extremity metastasis who appear to have a somewhat better prognosis (Wedin et al. 1999; Baloch et al. 2000) (Figure 14.4).

As stated, renal metastases tend to be very vascular. When curettage is preferred to *en bloc* excision, embolisation should be considered before surgical intervention (Figure 14.3), particularly if the lesion is in the spine, pelvis or proximal limb (Sun & Lang 1998; Layalle et al. 1998). It is our experience that embolisation before surgery significantly reduces intra-operative blood loss.

Palliative amputation is rarely indicated, but may be appropriate in painful fungating tumours of the lower leg where there are no remaining treatment options. Counselling of patient and relatives is essential to explain the rationale for treatment.

(a)

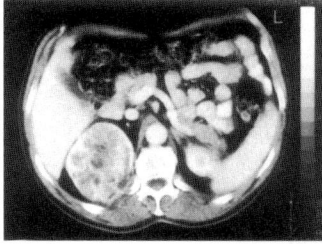

(b)

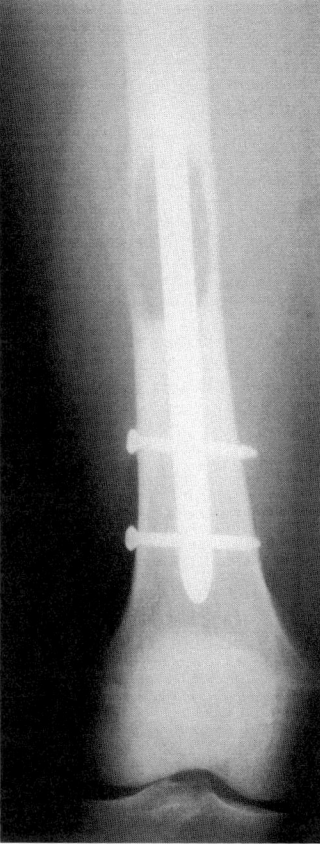

(c)

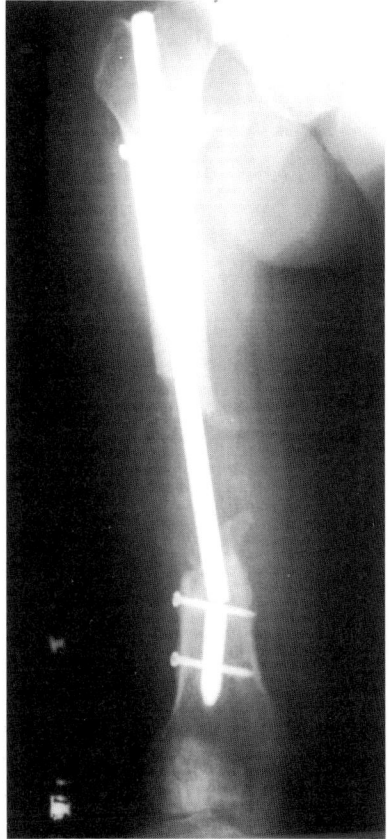

Figure 14.4 This patient with a renal cell carcinoma (a) had a single bony metastasis in the right femoral diaphysis (b). After nephrectomy, the patient had prophylactic intramedullary fixation. The patient survived longer than anticipated, the lesion increased significantly in size and the fixation failed (c). The patient went on to have an endoprosthetic replacement of the distal femur.

Regional surgery

Pelvis

Lesions in the pelvis may be very large. Reconstruction is challenging and may be inappropriate in advanced cases where stable fixation is unlikely to be achieved. Preoperative embolisation should be considered in all cases. Curettage followed by internal fixation and packing with bone cement is often the most appropriate treatment. If the hip joint is painful, involved by tumour or at risk of collapse, then acetabular reconstruction with internal fixation using screws and threaded rods to obtain fixation in the remaining good bone of the ilium, and cement augmentation coupled with total hip replacement, is indicated. This technique is generally referred to as the 'Harrington Procedure' (Harrington 1995). *En bloc* resection of pelvic tumours is rarely done as the morbidity is significant, and clear surgical margins are unlikely to be achieved. In solitary pelvic lesions, therefore, we would recommend the Harrington procedure with post-operative radiotherapy.

Proximal femur

Internal fixation of hip fractures should be avoided as the risk of implant failure is high, and stable fixation is rarely achieved because of bone destruction. The patient is likely therefore to be left with a painful unstable fixation that does not permit full weight bearing, and a probable requirement for further surgery. Femoral neck lesions may be adequately treated using cemented total hip arthroplasty or hemiarthroplasty. The risk of increased haemorrhage must be considered. Where there is extensive destruction extending into the intertrochanteric and subtrochanteric region, the preferred treatment is by *en bloc* resection and endoprosthetic replacement using custom or modular implants as used for primary bone tumours. The cost of such implants is recovered within a very short time if a previously immobile patient can be mobilised and discharged from hospital with no requirement for further surgery. (Chan et al. 1992; Capanna et al. 1999) (Figure 14.4).

Femoral diaphysis

Where there is a solitary diaphyseal lesion, endoprosthetic replacement should be considered. Small lesions with relatively little bone destruction can be successfully treated by locked intramedullary nailing, with or without curettage of the lesion followed by cement packing. Nailing of a lesion where there is a major bone defect is unlikely to achieve either mechanical stability or pain relief.

Distal femur/proximal tibia

En bloc resection of the lesion and endoprosthetic replacement is the preferred treatment (Figure 14.5). Small lesions may be treated by curettage and internal fixation with cement augmentation.

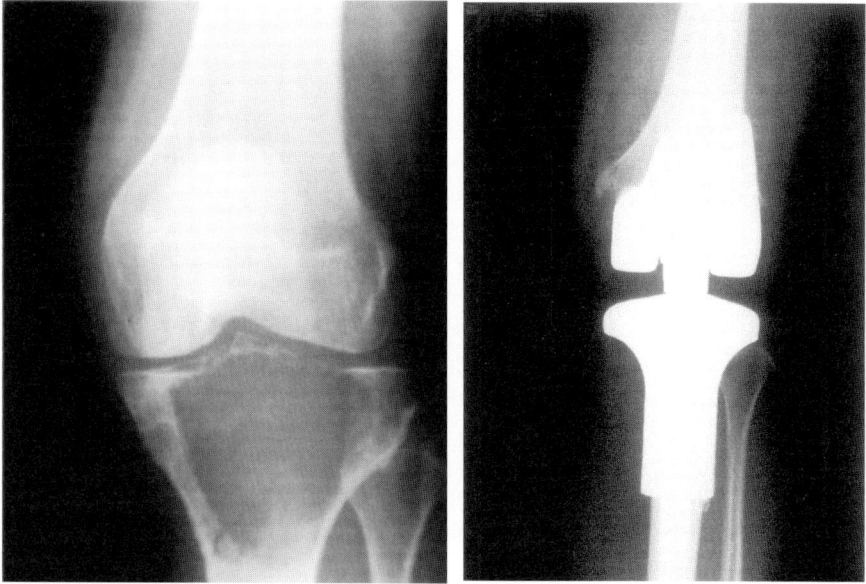

Figure 14.5 A patient with a solitary renal metastasis to the proximal tibia (a) was treated by en bloc resection and endoprosthetic replacement (b).

Humerus

Surgical principles for proximal lesions are similar to those outlined above for the proximal femur. Large solitary lesions are best treated by using an endoprosthesis. Other lesions may be treated with curettage followed by internal fixation with cement augmentation. A locked intramedullary nail is preferred for diaphyseal lesions.

Renal metastases may occur in many other sites, and treatment should be based around the four key issues discussed earlier.

When to involve the orthopaedic surgeon?

Ideally every cancer centre should have a multidisciplinary team. One member of this team should be an orthopaedic surgeon with a special interest in metastatic bone disease. All patients with bone pathology should be assessed by the lead clinician for metastatic bone disease so that appropriate intervention can be done at the earliest possible stage (Table 14.2). The temptation to perform immediate fixation by the on-call trauma team should be resisted. Specialised techniques are required for surgery on renal metastases and there is a learning curve for performing these procedures. Although there is no merit in undue delay, pre-operative planning and the use of appropriate techniques by an experienced surgical team are more important than speed of surgery. In the absence of such a team set-up, it is wise to seek orthopaedic advice in any patient with persisting pain, progressive bone changes, or a Mirels (1989) score of 8 or above (Table 14.1).

Table 14.2 Recommended referral for patients with renal cell carcinoma, who present to a urological surgeon

	Refer to:
Solitary bone lesion	Orthopaedic oncology surgeon
Multiple bone lesions	Oncologist
Impending or pathological fracture	Orthopaedic oncology surgeon

Conclusion

Renal metastases are uncommon, but important, as they appear to have a better prognosis than other metastatic bone tumours. As such, full multidisciplinary assessment is essential to come to an accurate diagnosis and to initiate adequate treatment.

Renal cell metastases respond relatively poorly to both chemotherapy and radiotherapy. Therefore, surgical stabilisation of skeletal metastases is essential to provide adequate pain relief and prevent pathological fractures.

Indications for urgent referral include an impending or actual pathological fracture. Large osteolytic lesions of weight-bearing bones that are painful are likely to fracture, and urgent referral to an orthopaedic oncologist is indicated for consideration of surgical stabilisation. Mirels scoring system (Table 14.1) can be helpful in assessing the risk of pathological fracture in an individual patient.

In our view, radical surgery can be justified in selected patients with solitary renal metastases, but there is an associated morbidity. Before embarking on radical surgery, it is essential that the patient's medical condition is optimised, that hypercalcaemia is corrected, and that embolisation is considered where appropriate.

Obviously, such radical treatment is not indicated in widespread disease and a more conservative approach should be adopted. Whenever orthopaedic intervention takes place, the aim should be to provide immediate and stable fixation, which will return the patient to as near a normal state as possible and which will outlast the expected survival time of that individual. Anything less will not be in the best interests of the patient concerned.

References

Baloch KG, Grimer RJ, Carter SR, Tillman RM (2000) Radical surgery for the solitary bony metastasis from renal cell carcinoma. *Journal of Bone and Joint Surgery (Br)*: **82-B**: 62–67.

Batson OV (1940) The function of the vertebral veins and their role in the spread of metastases. *Annals of Surgery* **112**: 138.

Capanna R, Campanacci D, Martelli L, Michels S, Bacci G (1999) The treatment of metastases in bone. In *European instructional course lectures* (ed. Jakob RP, Fulford P, Horan F), volume 4, pp. 24–34. London: EFFORT.

Chan D, Carter SR, Grimer RJ, Sneath RS (1992) Endoprosthetic replacement for bony metastases. *Annals of the Royal College of Surgeons of England* **74**: 13–18.

Cool P & Grimer RJ (2000) Pathological fractures of the extremities. *Trauma* **2**: 101–111.

de Kernion JB, Ramming KP, Smith RB (1978) The natural history of metastatic renal cell carcinoma: a computer analysis. *Journal of Urology* **120**:148–152.

Dineen MK, Pastore RD, Emrich LJ, Huben RP (1988) Results of surgical treatment of renal cell carcinoma with solitary metastasis. *Journal of Urology* **140**: 277–279.

Galasko CS & Sylvester BS (1978) Back pain in patients treated for malignant tumours. *Clinical Oncology* **4**: 273–283.

Harrington KD (1988) *Orthopaedic management of metastatic bone disease.* St Louis, Washington, Toronto: Mosby.

Harrington KD (1995) Orthopaedic management of extremity and pelvic lesions. *Clinical Orthopedics* **312**:136–147.

Hipp JA, Springfield DS, Hayes WC (1995) Predicting pathologic fracture risk in the management of metastatic bone defects. *Clinical Orthopedics* **312**: 120–135.

Huguenin PU, Kieser S, Glanzmann C, Capaul R, Lutolf UM (1998) Radiotherapy for metastatic carcinomas of the kidney or melanomas: an analysis using palliative end points. *International Journal of Radiation Oncology, Biology, Physics* **41**: 401–405.

Layalle I, Flandroy P, Trotteur G, Dondelinger RF (1998) Arterial embolization of bone metastases: is it worthwhile? *Journal Belge de Radiolgie* **81**: 223–225.

Maldazys JD & de Kernion JB (1986) Prognostic factors in metastatic renal carcinoma. *Journal of Urology* **136**: 376–379.

Mankin HJ, Lange TA, Spanier SS (1982) The hazards of biopsy in patients with malignant primary bone and soft tissue tumours. *Journal of Bone and Joint Surgery* **64**: 1121–1127.

Middleton RG (1967) Surgery for metastatic renal cell carcinoma. *Journal of Urology* **97**: 973–977.

Mirels H (1989) Metastatic disease in long bones. *Clinical Orthopedics* **249**: 256–264.

Montie JE, Stewart BH, Straffon RA et al. (1977) The role of adjunctive nephrectomy in patients with metastatic renal cell carcinoma. *Journal of Urology* **117**: 272–275.

O'Dea MJ, Zincke H, Utz DC, Bernatz PE (1978) The treatment of renal cell carcinoma with solitary metastasis. *Journal of Urology* **120**: 540–542.

Pongracz N, Zimmerman R, Kotz R (1988) Orthopaedic management of bony metastases of renal cancer. *Seminars in Surgical Oncology* **4**: 139–142.

Robbins SG, Lane JM, Healey JH, Cornell CN (1993) Metastatic bone disease: epidemiology, biology, diagnosis, and treatment. In *Diagnosis and management of pathological fractures* (ed. Lane JM & Healey JH), pp. 83–98. New York: Raven Press Ltd.

Stener B, Henriksson C, Johansson S, Gunterberg B, Petterson S (1984) Surgical removal of bone and muscle metastases of renal cancer. *Acta Orthopaedica Scandinavica* **55**: 491–500.

Sun S & Lang EV (1998) Bone metastases from renal cell carcinoma: preoperative embolisation. *Journal of Vascular and Interventional Radiology* **9**: 263–269.

Tillman RM (1999) The role of the orthopaedic surgeon in metastatic disease of the appendicular skeleton. *Journal of Bone and Joint Surgery (Br)* **81-B**: 1–2.

Tolia BM & Whitmore WF (1975) Solitary metastasis from renal cell carcinoma. *Journal of Urology* **114**: 836–838.

Tongaonkar HB, Kulkarni JN, Kamat MR (1992) Solitary metastases from renal cell carcinoma: a review. *Journal of Surgical Oncology* **49**: 45–48.

Wedin R, Bauer HCF, Wersall P (1999) Failures after operations for skeletal metastatic lesions of long bones. *Clinical Orthopaedics and Related Research* **358**: 128–139.

PART 6

Clinical governance and service development

Auditing the quality of services for the investigation and management of renal cell carcinoma: the growing importance of formal accreditation and appraisal

Nicholas D James and D Mike A Wallace

Introduction

The increasing prominence of clinical outcome data, linked to revalidation and clinical governance, has focused attention on the problem of how to collect clinical data. Two different large audits are highlighted in this article: one performed by the Section of Oncology of the British Association of Urology Surgeons (BAUS), the other by The Royal College of Radiologists (RCR). Both audits show wide variations in practice and in numbers treated per centre, and illustrate potentially complementary ways of obtaining rapid, good quality, comparative clinical data. If clinical governance is ever to be really credible, good quality comparative data are essential but hard to obtain. Frequently, data collection is patchy, uses inconsistent methodology, is done too late to be of great value or is inconsistently coded. There are also substantial logistical constraints on collecting clinical data sets in busy clinical settings.

Two data collection methods were used: the traditional paper form and an online method. Paper-based collection is simple and requires no special equipment but also is time consuming and often inconsistent. Electronic data collection has several potential advantages. Multiple data re-entry may be reduced by electronic transfer of completed data forms. Data entry can be constrained to relevant items by multiple-choice lists, supported by drop-down 'Help' screens.

Having collected data, some form of analysis must be performed and interpretation put upon the data. If possible, the collected data should be used to underpin changes in practice in the future, and also as a tool for further audits to monitor changes in outcome consequent on any changes in practice.

Methods
BAUS data collection

The BAUS Section of Oncology has run a registry of newly presenting urological tumours since 1 January 1999, collecting a minimum dataset applicable to all tumours. This minimum dataset can be collected on a paper form and sent electronically or by mail. From 1999 to 2002, the percentage of participating centres using electronic data submission has increased to 61.7%. In 2000, 356 consultants in 154 hospital centres submitted data on 24,343 newly presenting urological cancers to the BAUS Section of Oncology, where the data have been analysed. Of these cancers, 2037 were renal carcinomas. The minimum dataset consists of questions on demography, referral, clinical and pathological staging, and initial management. Figure 15.1 shows the age and sex distribution of these cases.

RCR data collection

All radiotherapy centres in the UK were contacted and asked to provide details on 50 consecutive patients who had completed radiotherapy before the date of inception of the survey. This number of patients spanned different time intervals in different centres dependent on overall workload, but it was felt necessary to allow a representative overview of practice in each centre.

The following items were recorded for each radiotherapy centre: NHS Trust Name, to which a standard code was automatically linked; Trust policy for planned interruptions (e.g. machine service days, public holidays); Trust policy for unplanned interruptions (e.g. machine breakdown, patient toxicity). These data items were completed once. For the patients, the following items collected are given in Table 15.1. The online tool is illustrated in Figure 15.2.

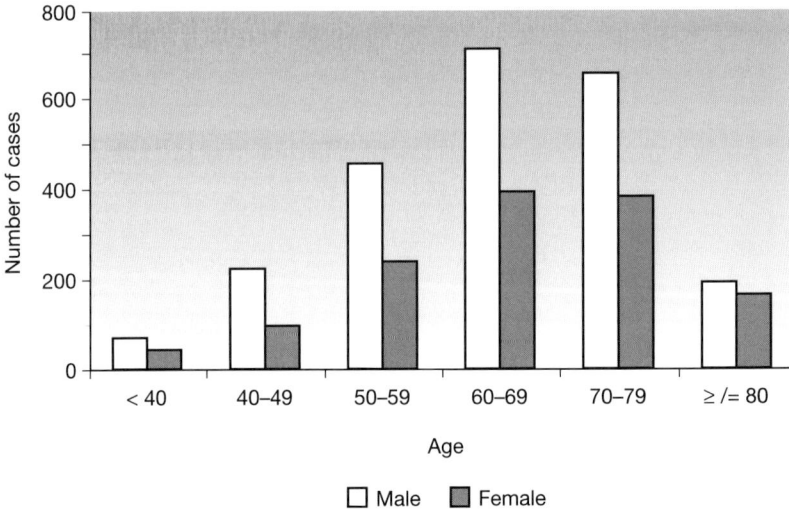

Figure 15.1 Age and sex distribution of renal carcinoma cases in the BAUS audit diagnosis

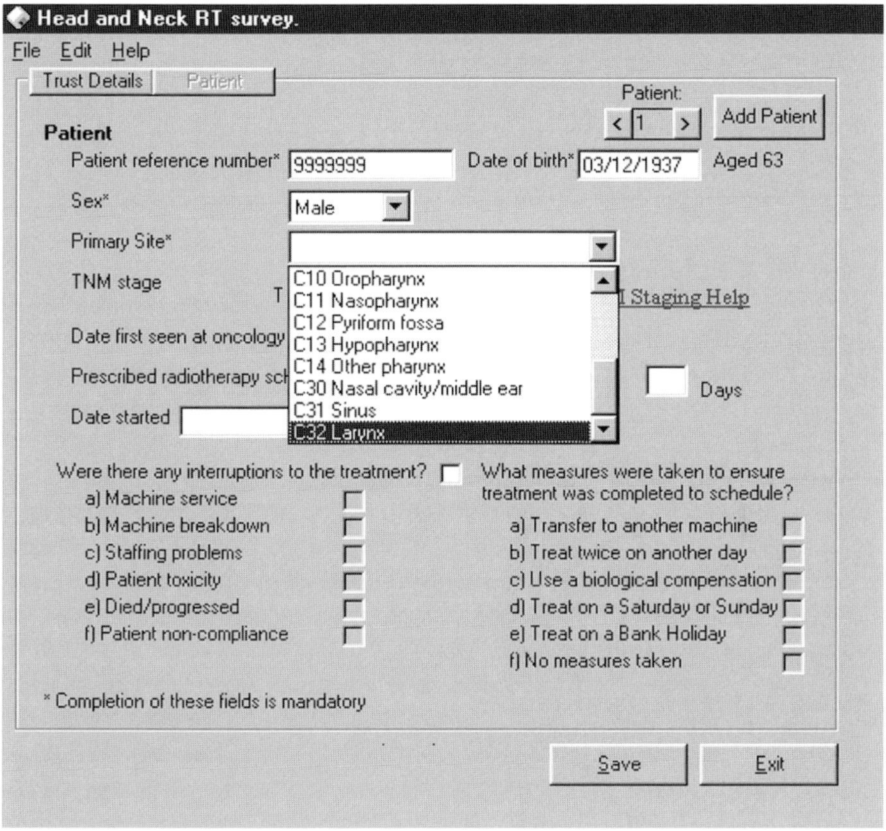

Figure 15.2 Specimen screen shot from radiotherapy audit

Results

Table 15.1 shows the number of tumours for the three main urology sites broken down by consultant. As can readily be seen, there is a very wide variation, with a very low median number of renal tumours per consultant compared with prostate and bladder cancer. Nonetheless, a few consultants treat large numbers of renal tumours each year. Table 15.2 shows the stage breakdown and numbers of renal cancer patients treated. This amounts to 41% of the total UK incidence for the same period (see Chapter One). Figure 15.1 shows the age and sex distribution of cases. The age and sex mix are typical of other published series but have a younger age than the comparable figures from the UK cancer intelligence units, which recorded 4996 cases for the UK in 1997. This validates the quality of data collection for this item and also gives a broad baseline snapshot of patterns of presentation in the UK. The stage mix will form a valuable baseline for future studies and may change in the future: in Germany, for example, there is a much higher usage of abdominal

Table 15.1 Tumours per consultant

Organ	Total number	Median	Range
Prostate	12,892	29	0–155
Bladder	7549	17	0–84
Kidney	2037	4	0–46

Table 15.2 Stage distribution at diagnosis

Stage I	614 (33%)
Stage II	424 (23.5%)
Stage III	449 (24.7%)
Stage IV	328 (18%) of which 215 (11.8%) M1

ultrasound in primary care and innovations such as this may alter the presenting stage mix.

For the renal cancers 47.9% were referred by general practitioners and 36.7% by other hospital practitioners. These percentages are the lowest and highest for all the urological cancers, reflecting the wide spectrum of presentation of this tumour. Only 75% of renal cancers were treated with curative intent and 14.6% had no histological confirmation of renal cancer, diagnosis being made mainly by radiology.

Table 15.3 shows the initial intent of treatment for the renal tumours treated, broken down by broad treatment category. Organ-conserving- or nephron-sparing surgery was done on only 61 cases. These operations were done in only 32 centres, which performed between 1–8 such operations. 1173 radical nephrectomies were done with curative intent, and 121 with palliative intent. It seems likely that there is some mis-categorisation or else misplaced optimism: neither radiotherapy nor chemotherapy is realistically likely to cure patients, but a small proportion apparently received their treatments with curative intent. Nonetheless, the general picture that

Table 15.3 Initial treatment

Curative	1415 (75.2%)
Surveillance	111 (5.9%)
Palliative	356 (18.9%)

	Curative	Surveillance	Palliative
Radical surgery	1173	2	121
Organ conserving	60		1
Radiotherapy	11	1	33
ChemoRx	7	2	10
ImmunoRx	11	1	62

emerges is likely to be broadly accurate. What are lacking in these data are details of treatment for relapses, or indeed second-line treatment after, for example, initial surgery. Also, we may be underestimating the use of adjuvant treatments, particularly the use of adjuvant immunotherapy after surgery, as the decision to give this treatment may be made by an oncologist after the urologist has submitted the dataset of the patient to BAUS.

Figure 15.2 shows a typical screen shot from the RCR audit, illustrating the use of constrained lists and drop-down 'Help' boxes. Results of this audit have been published separately (James et al. 2002), and so only samples will be included here for purposes of illustration. Table 15.4 shows the overall number of cases collected. Altogether all bar one UK radiotherapy centre returned data sets on patients, mostly on the requested 50 consecutive cases. There is, of course, no way to validate whether the cases are consecutive or not but again a reasonably clear overview of patterns of care emerges.

Table 15.4 Summary results from radiotherapy audit

Number of centres	56/57
Patients	2620 patients (2.9:1 male:female)
Age mean	62.8, interquartile range 54–72 years

Discussion

These results show that it is possible to collect large amounts of data from busy clinicians in relatively short time periods. The BAUS data, however, only cover about half of the total incidence for the period. There are several possible reasons for this under-reporting. Firstly, not all cases of renal cancer will present to urologists who are members of BAUS and who are participants in the audit. Even if all urologists were to participate (around 70% do), not all cases of renal cancer will be seen by urologists: a minority will be seen by other surgical specialities or will present with, for example, metastatic disease to physicians. It would seem likely that a significant proportion of the cases not seen by urologists will end up with oncologists for treatment of metastatic diseases and thus joint inter-speciality audit may improve completeness of data capture. To explore this possibility, a joint BAUS/RCR audit of practice in muscle-invasive bladder cancer is currently being planned by the authors. The BAUS data are collected by surgeons who are likely to be sub-specialising in oncology and 'enthusiasts' as far as cancer treatment is concerned in that they are sufficiently motivated to take part in a national audit of their practice over and above other workload commitments. Moving towards joint data collection with the oncologists who constitute another important component of the multidisciplinary team would doubtless strengthen the data collection effort. It would also provide improved coverage of practice less well covered by the BAUS data such as treatment of relapsed disease. With the advent of the National Cancer Plan, the implementation of collection of the National Cancer Minimum Data Set is none the less going to present problems if good data are only obtainable on half of the treated patients.

Outcome data for the UK also show worse outcomes when compared with other European countries and the USA. This may partly reflect patterns in diagnosis, for example the wider availability of office ultrasound in Germany, but it is also likely to reflect differences in treatment. For bladder and prostate cancer, both much commoner, there are moves to limit radical operations to surgeons performing a pre-set minimum of operations each year. At present, there are no such moves to limit kidney operations in the same fashion, despite smaller numbers of patients per consultant (Table 15.1). Furthermore, although a radical nephrectomy is a relatively straightforward procedure, there are several improvements on this technique that are very much within the domain of the 'super-specialist' only. These range from less morbid procedures such as partial nephrectomy or laparoscopic nephrectomy for good prognosis tumours through to supra-radical procedures for patients with IVC extension or penetration of the renal capsule or nodal involvement. With the appearance of data justifying nephrectomy in the presence of metastatic disease and immunotherapy for advanced disease, the referral of these patients to specialist centres also becomes necessary. This leaves a decreasing number of patients with a relatively rare tumour being managed in non-specialist centres, making it increasingly difficult to justify not referring all such patients to the centre. A possible route around this concentration of all patients in the centre is proposed in Tables 15.5–15.7.

Table 15.5 Who should manage which cases?

'Standard' cases	Complex cases
≥ = 5 nephrectomies per year	Large MDT
MDT	Nephrology/dialysis
Radiology	Cardiothoracic surgery and ITU
Oncology	Specialist radiology
Pathology	Hepatobiliary surgery
Specialist nurses	Vascular surgery
	Oncology

Table 15.6 How to optimise decision making?

Standard cases managed in cancer units
Complex cases managed in specialist centre
Potentially complex cases presenting to cancer units to be discussed at cancer centre MDT

Table 15.7 Definitions of standard and complex cases

Complex cases	Standard cases
Nephron sparing surgery indicated	All cases not falling in first column
IVC involvement	
Locally advanced: T4 or N+	
Metastatic disease	
Renal impairment	
Multiple/ bilateral tumours	

Patients with complex features require a broader scope of specialist inputs (Table 15.5). Potentially complex cases presenting in cancer units can be 'filtered' via the multidisciplinary team (MDT) in the cancer centre, and an agreed management plan proposed. Table 15.7 gives a possible classification of complex and standard cases.

Conclusion

The good clinical governance of renal cell carcinoma services is integrally dependant upon the routine collection of high quality clinical data based on the monitoring of evidence-based clinical guidelines and care pathways for effective investigation and management. The current chapter provides some insights into how suitable systems may be set up within the clinical setting in order to ensure that adequate information relating to the care of patients with RCC is available to the MDT for continuous review.

Recommended reading

Anderson J, Oliver RTD & Miles A (Eds). The Effective Management of Urological Malignacy. Aesculapius Medical Press. London 2004.

Berk M, Callaly T & Hyland M. The evolution of clinical audit as a tool for quality improvement. *Journal of Evaluation in Clinical Practice* **9**, 251–257.

James R & Miles A (Eds). Managed Care Networks: principles and practice. Aesculapius Medical Press. London 2002.

Johnston G. Crombie IK, Davies HTO, Alder EM & Millard A (2000) Reviewing audit: barriers and facilitating factors for effective clinical audit. *Quality in Health Care* **9**, 23–36.

Miles A & Lugon M (Eds). Effective Clinical Practice. Blackwell Science Ltd. Oxford 1996.

Miles A, Grey JE, Polychronis A, Price N & Melchiorri C (2004) Developments in the evidence-based health care debate – 2004. *Journal of Evaluation in Clinical Practice* **10**, 129–142.

McNulty T & Ferlie E. Re-engineering health care. University Press. Oxford 2002.

Chapter 16

Learning about cancer: initial findings from a study of the acceptability and usefulness of the web as a cancer information resource

Harry Daniels, Jan Derry, Rubina Rahman, Annie Young and Nicholas James

Two in five of the UK population will develop cancer during their lifetime and one in four will die from it; the majority of the population is therefore affected either as a patient, or as a friend, relative or carer, and will therefore have a need for information about the disease (Department of Health 1999). Cancer patients use different information sources and media as their disease progresses (Butow et al. 1997). There appear to be benefits for different groups of all media types on measures of, for example, knowledge, anxiety and depression (Devine et al. 1995; Mohide et al. 1996). Carers assiduously pursue information as part of the process of caring for and supporting patients (Derdrian 1989). There is also evidence to suggest that more quality information can lead to better outcomes in the treatment of cancer. However, many patients with cancer are unhappy about the amount of information that they receive from their doctors, and are critical of the manner in which the diagnosis is delivered or how diagnostic procedures and treatment options are discussed.

In this chapter we present an interim report of a study of patients' and carers' use of, attitudes to and beliefs about the web as a cancer information source. Although the focus of the study is the relative efficacy of the web compared with other sources of information, it is predicted that findings will be generalisable in most respects to other diseases or conditions. The expectation is that the study will result in findings specific to the internet and also in better understanding of its complementary functions in relation to the range of information resources available to the general public. In this context we introduce our approach to theorising processes of learning about cancer.

Inequalities in health

Inequalities in health have been well publicised since the Black Report (Black et al. 1980). The current government has committed itself to reducing such inequalities. The NHS Plan introduced a national 'inequalities target' with cancer as one of three clinical priorities. However, their determinants of inequality are complex and deeply ingrained in our social structure. People from deprived and less affluent backgrounds are more likely to get some types of cancer and overall are more likely to die from it once it has been diagnosed (Selby 1996). In the early 1990s, deaths from lung cancer among men were nearly five times higher among unskilled workers than among professional groups (Butow et al. 1997). Similarly, Loehrer et al. (1991) found that Americans living in poverty experience a higher incidence of and greater mortality from cancer than the 'non-poor'. At least 50% of the difference in mortality was believed to be caused by a delay in diagnosis, although risk-promoting lifestyles and behaviours also contributed to poorer survival. A potential exacerbating factor among the poor was thought to be inadequate information and knowledge about cancer and its treatment. Their findings suggest that misinformation and misconceptions regarding cancer and its treatment among patients contributes to inappropriate care-seeking behaviours.

There is a paucity of UK and European literature on clinical outcomes for minority ethnic cancer patients. The few studies that have been completed have shown that minority ethnic groups have significantly poorer cure rates for some cancers and that diagnosis at a more advanced stage is one of the causal factors. However, white cancer patients have been found to have better survival than black cancer patients *even when matched* for the stage of disease found at diagnosis and age (Barker and Baker 1990; Muir 1996). Inequity in *access* to health services has been noted frequently (Acheson Report 1998). This is not restricted to social class and geography; people in minority ethnic communities are less likely to receive the services they need. Women from these groups do not come forward for breast and cervical screening. Culturally sensitive information and different approaches to giving information can often improve the accessibility to screening to these groups (Butow et al. 1997). However, as Pfeffer and Moynihan (1996) report, none of the investigations into health beliefs with respect to cancer has set out to investigate the significance of ethnicity alone.

The current study

Our interests lie in information seeking, particularly among ethnic minority cancer patients and those patients living in poverty. The study we report here seeks to establish:

- what attributes of information resources are important for patients and carers
- which attributes of information resources are associated with particular media types
- which media types are associated with success in finding useful information
- differences in use, attitudes and beliefs about the web associated with cancer site
- differences in use, attitudes and beliefs about the web associated with demographic factors, internet experience and patient or carer status.

The study is being carried out in three Birmingham teaching hospitals: a cancer centre, serving the West Midlands region, and two inner city general hospitals with cancer units closely linked to the main cancer centre which serve areas with large ethnic minority populations and significant social deprivation. It is a two-phase study.

For phase 1, data collection instruments have been developed through interviews. A purposive sample was recruited, consisting of patients with the specific cancers and carers with a range of demographic characteristics and different experiences of use of information resources.

One of the strengths of this study is that it investigates users' attitudes, beliefs and practices through survey items derived from non-directive methods of elicitation. Participant involvement, motivation and feedback have been taken into consideration in the project design. Two non-directive methods for interviewing have been used to establish the items for the questionnaire. The principal method is derived from personal construct theory; this has been supplemented by use of a nominal group technique. Data from interviews have been analysed using data reduction and portrayal techniques, in which categories of constructs were successively induced, applied, refined and reapplied (Miles and Huberman 1994).

Individual interviews were held to determine personal constructs relating to cancer information resources using a technique derived from personal construct analysis (Bannister and Fransella 1989). The 'elements' were obtained by asking patients to list ways of getting information about cancer, e.g. video, TV, leaflet, website, doctor. The next stage requires participants to establish 'contrasts' between the elements by identifying similarities and differences between them. The descriptors they produced were used to generate 'constructs' by inviting respondents to indicate an opposite to each descriptor, e.g. 'cheap–expensive', 'familiar–new', 'specific–general', etc. Using repertory grids, interviewees were then invited to give a rating for the construct to show how well it describes each of the elements (Smith 1995).

The nominal group technique encourages maximum contributions from all group members, promotes idea generation, brainstorming and participation, and fosters tolerance of conflicting ideas. This technique assumes that the more ideas are generated, the greater the likelihood that superior ideas will emerge. The procedure is as follows:

1   Individuals generate ideas during or before the group meeting.
2   Each person takes a turn reading one of their ideas and ideas are written in a central place until all are listed.
3   The group discusses the ideas, possibly adding ideas to the list.
4   Each group member ranks the listed ideas.
5   Individual rankings are summarised for each idea to form a group ranking.
6   The group ranking of ideas is discussed.
7   If the group ranking is unacceptable, steps 3–6 are repeated (Chapple and Murphy 1996).

On the basis of our study of preferences for different sources of information (James et al. 1999), the provisional hypothesis of this study is that the web will not be more highly valued overall than other types of resources (including health professionals), but that it will be more highly valued for certain characteristics or properties (e.g. controllability, being up to date, interactivity and anonymity). However, the purpose of basing this study on personal constructs was to elicit participant attitudes about which we may not yet be aware.

The data gathered in this way generated topics for exploration in phase 2. Findings suggest the following:

- The diversity of sources of information used by patients and carers correlates with social class.
- Different information needs are articulated by patients as a function of their age.
- Carers are more likely to engage with the internet than patients.
- The type and stage of disease conditions, information-seeking behaviour as well as availability of information (e.g. availability of specialist support in the case of breast cancer).
- Patients place different value on specific professional information sources (e.g. nurses tend to be valued for their general care and concern rather than the detailed information that is provided by clinicians).
- Patients distinguished between information sources that they regarded as oriented to choice or compliance. They felt that some sources were designed to persuade rather than inform.
- Patients distinguished between those services with a consumer as against a provider orientation. They felt that they had no options or choices in provider-oriented services.
- The modality through which the information was presented was discussed in terms of the characteristics of use that it allowed (e.g. whether it was possible to revisit, check [quality and memory] and interrogate the source) as well as the affective conditions in which information was relayed (e.g. sympathetic, in prompted dialogue)

Further analysis of the data is required to substantiate these initial suggestions. However, the following three matters featured widely: ethnicity and health beliefs, sex and information sources.

Ethnicity and health beliefs

Two of the cancer sites serve large areas with large ethnic minority populations and significant social deprivation. As a result many other issues began to emerge, regarding minority ethnic groups and their information-seeking behaviour.

Qualitative data revealed that traditional beliefs exist and that there are also contrasting attitudes whereby many patients and carers hold on to their cultural beliefs. This can have an effect on the patients' or carers' information-seeking behaviour, and in particular the use of the web. Observation and interviews with members from minority ethnic groups revealed that information-seeking behaviour was non-existent among this group.

Many first-generation working class Bangladeshi and Pakistani patients talked about cancer being the will of 'Allah' (God) and that seeking information from other sources would be of no help.

> . . . no amount of knowledge can help me now. Reading a book or looking on the computer will not help what is the will of Allah . . .
>
> A first-generation Pakistani breast cancer patient

> . . . I don't think that looking for more information is good . . . the doctor knows my case and tells me what I need to know, how can I know more than the doctor . . .

> I wouldn't know where to look . . . what has happened to me is in Allah's hands now.
>
> A first-generation Pakistani carer whose son has cancer

Sex

The fieldwork observations revealed that women patients and carers valued the knowledge derived from information seeking more than men. They tended to use more categories of coping strategies (e.g. family support, friends' support and religious support). It appeared that the working class men in our sample generally felt uncomfortable about seeking further information and finding out more.

Once they left the clinic, they preferred a policy of life as normal in which cancer could be forgotten. As one male patient with bladder cancer receiving chemotherapy revealed in a personal construct interview:

> . . . once I am out of here I'm gonna forget I've got it . . . I don't need to find out anything else or read no books all I need is to get through each day normally like everyone else . . .

In contrast a breast patient reveals:

> . . . I needed to find out as much as I could . . . I went to the library, I always talking to the other patients when I was in chemo . . . and I always have a set of questions ready before I see the doctor . . .

Information sources

Personal construct interviews revealed that patients used a variety of other sources of information. The main contrasts were their perceptions of general vs specific information. The following quotes will illustrate this further.

> . . . leaflets are really useful at the beginning cause they don't give too much information which can scare you to death, books are more detailed and you can find out more about tumours . . .
>
> A 45-year-old breast cancer patient of black origin

> . . .I don't understand no books cause they've got too much detail, leaflets are easy cause they are general . . .
>
> A 61-year-old male colorectal patient of white origin

Discussion and conclusion: learning about cancer

In addition to the specific matters noted above, we became very aware of the need to develop an account of learning about cancer within our study.

Fallowfield and Jenkins (1999) reported that many patients leave consultations unsure about the diagnosis and prognosis, confused about the meaning of – and need for – further diagnostic tests, unclear about the management plan and uncertain about the true therapeutic intent of treatment. In addition, communication difficulties may impede the recruitment of patients to clinical trials, delaying the introduction of efficacious new treatments into clinics. Although it is recognised that communicating about cancer and death is a major challenge, research suggests that this is even greater where language and culture differ (Cancer Support Centre 2000).

We argue that it is beneficial and appropriate to analyse social practices of health information seeking and providing as components of an educational practice. Recent analyses of educational practice have emphasised the sociocultural nature of the activity (Daniels 2001). Wood and Wood (1996a, 1996b) and Wood (1998) have developed an approach to tutoring that is based on an interpretation of Vygotsky's (1987) notion of the 'zone of proximal development' (ZPD). The concept of ZPD was created by Vygotsky as a metaphor to assist in explaining the way in which social and participatory learning takes place: the ZPD is defined as the difference between the 'actual developmental level as determined by independent problem solving' and the higher level of 'potential development as determined through problem solving under adult guidance or in collaboration with more capable peers'.

The two principles of *uncertainty* and *contingency* form the central features of the Wood and Wood approach. It is suggested that uncertainty makes learning more difficult. When a learner is uncertain or unfamiliar with the relevant features of a task, motivation, task orientation and memory of the task itself are reduced. This suggestion echoes that of Greeno's (1991) concerning 'learning the landscape' of a task or task environment. For Greeno, an expert is, in part, someone who has is familiar with the task terrain, its features and demands. Thus, an expert is someone who has reduced the uncertainty in a task situation. Learners for whom uncertainty is high require support in the process of reducing the uncertainty or 'learning the landscape' of the task. The second key principle of the approach is that support offered within the ZPD of a learner whose uncertainty about a task is high is that it (the support) should be *contingent* upon the responses of the learner. The notions of *uncertainty*, *contingency* and learning the knowledge *landscape* may be applied to processes of learning about cancer.

A diagnosis of cancer is a psychologically distressing event and affects the patient's ability to absorb and remember information. They become more *uncertain*. These attitudes are reflected in the efforts that patients make to obtain further information, or to resist further information that is offered to them. However a diagnosis of cancer may invoke fear, and loss of self-esteem, and this can sometimes be alleviated by information (Butow et al. 1997). Lack of information can increase uncertainty, anxiety, distress, and dissatisfaction. One study revealed that the level of psychological distress in patients with serious illness is less when they think they have received adequate information (Fallowfield et al. 1990). On the basis of a very large sample, Jenkins et al. (2001) provide conclusive evidence that the vast majority of patients with cancer want a great deal of specific information about their illness and treatment, i.e. they want information that is *contingent* upon their specific needs. This suggests that information seeking should be supported in such a way that information that is contingent on need may be found. In a complex knowledge domain such as knowledge about cancer, there is a need for some form of 'expert' help for novices who are attempting to learn the knowledge *landscape* of their disease in order to identify *contingent* information that will help reduce their *uncertainty*. Such an 'expert' has to be effective in a variety of contexts. Green and Leydon (2001) have studied how doctors and their patients make the consultation 'work' but had not designed their study with a specific focus on ethnic minority groups.

Brown et al. (1999) have shown that a minor adjustment in the social practice of consultation can be effective. They conclude that a question prompt sheet addressed by the doctor is a simple, inexpensive and effective means of promoting patient question asking in the cancer consultation. In the context of innovative health technology (IHT) use, Gentile (1998) showed that a more sophisticated (expert) user such as the oncology professional will more likely help the patient to learn about the knowledge *landscape* of the disease. Pergament et al. (1999) argued that the appropriate and effective use of the internet is rapidly expanding in medicine and that patterns of use are likely to co-evolve with changes in patient–healthcare provider relationships. They outlined steps that clinical oncologists and other healthcare professionals can take to direct and control the potential of the internet so as to optimise patient care. Each of these strategies requires health professionals to be proactive and sensitive in their engagement with their patients' processes of learning.

We have been piloting changes in our delivery of information based on the study findings as well as those of Pergament and Gentile. Patients seen in the joint urological clinic frequently need to be referred from the surgical to the non-surgical side, e.g. for consideration of radiotherapy. Patients are sent to the information room with a recommended list of pages and sections of the Cancer-Help UK website (www. cancerhelp.org.uk) to visit. The room contains an internet terminal dedicated for patient use and supported by volunteers. If desired, they can print out the suggested pages to read either before the consultation or at a later date. The professional selection of relevant pages helps users navigate the unfamiliar 'landscape' and maximises both clinician time and the time of the volunteers in the information room. We have previously shown (Tweddle et al. 2000) that patients from all backgrounds can successfully navigate web-based information given initial tuition. Nevertheless, many patients prefer to have help in navigation. This system gives individually tailored patient information and is very popular with patients because they feel that they have been given a very personal service. The use of a well-written website in this context maximises the benefits of the web and minimises the need to write, print and update local information sources. Where 'holes' in the website are identified (e.g. tips for coping with interferon therapy), locally produced information was incorporated into the website material (NJ is Editor in Chief of the site). By working with a familiar site, there are thus benefits for healthcare staff, patients and also the information provider. This preliminary experience suggests that to maximise the benefit of web-based information, websites must work actively with their audiences to identify ways of optimising delivery of material beyond the boundaries of the computer screen and into the human users of the services.

Sadler et al. (1998) suggest that cultural, linguistic and economic barriers place many ethnic minority groups in jeopardy of missing opportunities for disease prevention, early diagnosis, prompt treatment and participation in clinical trials. Sung et al. (1997) report that a direct focus on knowledge is more effective than a focus on belief and attitude. Sadler et al. (1998) reported that the development of a demonstration health education and prevention programme involving hands-on teaching aids helped to overcome language and educational barriers. Huang et al. (1999) showed that providing information in a culturally sensitive manner could assist doctors in providing optimum care and support for ethnic minority groups.

Current research activity

On the basis of the data from phase 1 and our current review of the literature, a questionnaire was developed. The model of learning outlined above has informed the design of the instrument. The questionnaire probes views about the processes of learning about cancer alongside issues raised through the outcomes of phase 1 interviews.

Great care was taken in the development of the questionnaire. In total it was piloted four times with patients and carers. The final questionnaire contains a total of 35 questions including a mixture of open and closed questions and ranking scales. Each question was tested for reliability and validity with a selection of 62 patients/carers. We will report the findings in 2003.

References

Acheson Report (1998) *In Independent Inquiry into Inequalities in Health*. London: HMSO.
Bannister D, Fransella F (1989) *Inquiring Man: The Psychology of Personal Constructs*. London: Routledge.
Barker RM, Baker MR (1990) Incidence of cancer in Bradford Asians. *Journal of Epidemiology and Community Health* **44**: 125–129.
Black D et al. (1980) *Inequalities in Health: Report of the Research Working Group*. London: Department of Health and Social Security.

Brown R, Butow PN, Boyer MJ, Tattersall MH (1999) Promoting patient participation in the cancer consultation: evaluation of a prompt sheet and coaching in question asking. *British Journal of Cancer* **80**: 242–248.

Butow PN, Maclean M, Dunn SM, Tattersall MHN, Boyer MJ (1997) The dynamics of change: Cancer patients' preferences for information, involvement and support. *Annals of Oncology* **8**: 857–863.

Cancer Support Centre (2000) *Views and Experiences of Cancer Service Users in Bradford and District.* Bradford: Cancer Support Centre.

Chapple M, Murphy R (1996) The nominal group technique: extending the evaluation of students' teaching and learning experiences. *Assessment and Evaluation in Higher Education* **21**: 147–159.

Daniels H (2001) *Vygotsky and Pedagogy.* London: Routledge.

Department of Health (1999) *Saving Lives: Our Healthier Nation.* London: DoH.

Derdrian AK (1989) Effects of information on recently diagnosed cancer patients' and spouses' satisfaction with care. *Cancer Nursing* **12**: 285–292.

Devine EC, Westlake SK (1995) The effects of psychoeducational care provided to adults with cancer: meta-analysis of 116 studies. *Oncology Nursing Forum* **22**: 1369–1381.

Fallowfield L, Jenkins V (1999) Effective communication skills are the key to good cancer care. *European Journal of Cancer* **35**: 1592–1597.

Fallowfield L, Hall A, Maguire GP, Baum J (1990) Psychological outcomes of different treatment policies in women with cancer outside a clinical trial. *British Medical Journal* **301**: 575–578.

Gentile JA (1998) Databases, websites, and the Internet. *Oncology (Huntington)* **12**: 356–359.

Green J, Leydon GM (2001). The management of information in out patient oncology ESRC award R000223142.

Greeno J (1991) Number sense a situated knowing in a conceptual domain. *Journal for Research in Mathematics Education* **22**: 117–218.

Huang X, Butow P, Meiser B, Goldstein D (1999) Attitudes and information needs of Chinese migrant cancer patients and their relatives. *Australian and New Zealand Journal of Medicine* **29**: 207–213.

James C, James N, Davies D, Harvey P, Tweddle S (1999) Preferences for different sources of information about cancer. *Patient Education and Counselling* in press.

Jenkins V, Fallowfield L, Saul J (2001) Information needs of patients with cancer: results from a large study in UK cancer centres. *British Journal of Cancer* **84**: 48–51.

Loehrer PJ, Greger HA, Weinberger M et al. (1991) Knowledge and beliefs about cancer in a socioeconomically disadvantaged population. *Cancer* **68**: 1665–1671.

Miles MB, Huberman AM (1994) *Qualitative Data Analysis: An expanded sourcebook*, 2nd edn. London: SAGE.

Mohide EA, Whelan TJ, Rath D et al. (1996) A randomised trial of two information packages distributed to new cancer patients before their initial appointment at a regional cancer centre. *British Journal of Cancer* **73**: 1588–1593.

Muir CS (1996) Epidemiology of cancer in ethnic groups. *British Journal of Cancer* **74**(suppl), S12–S16.

Pergament D, Pergament E, Wonderlick A, Fiddler M (1999) At the crossroads: the intersection of the Internet and clinical oncology. *Oncology (Huntington)* **13**: 577–583.

Pfeffer N, Moynihan P (1996) Ethnicity and health beliefs with respect to cancer: a critical review of methodology. *British Journal of Cancer* **74**(suppl): S66–S72.

Sadler GR, Nguyen F, Doan QAu, Thomas AG (1998) Strategies for reaching Asian Americans with health information. *American Journal of Preventive Medicine* **14**: 224–228.

Selby P (1996) Cancer clinical outcomes form minority ethnic groups. *British Journal of Cancer* **74**(suppl XXIX): S54–S60.

Smith JA (1995) Repertory grids: an interactive, case-study perspective. In: Smith JA, Harre R, Van Langenhove L (eds), *Rethinking Methods in Psychology*. London: Sage.

Sung JF, Blumenthal DS, Coates RJ, Alema-Mensah E (1997) Knowledge, beliefs, attitudes, and cancer screening among inner-city African-American women. *Journal of the National Medical Association* **89**: 405–411.

Tweddle S, James C, Daniels H, Davies D, Harvey P, James N, Mossman J, Woolf E (2000) Use of a web site for learning about cancer. *Computers and Education* **35**: 309–325.

Vygotsky LS (1987) *The Collected Works of L.S. Vygotsky,* vol. 1: *Problems of General Psychology*, including the volume *Thinking and Speech* (Rieber RW and Carton AS eds) (Minick N trans.). New York: Plenum Press.

Wood D (1998) *How Children Think and Learn: The social contexts of cognitive development.* Oxford: Blackwell Publishers Ltd.

Wood D, Wood H (1996a) Commentary: contingency in tutoring and learning. *Learning and Instruction*, **6**: 391–397.

Wood D, Wood H (1996b) Vygotsky, tutoring and learning. *Oxford Review of Education* **22**: 5–16.

Index